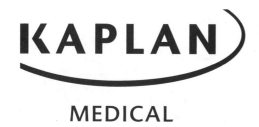

MEDICAL

USMLE®
Step 2 CS
Practice Cases
2020

Prep + Proven Strategies

© 2020 by Kaplan, Inc.

Published by Kaplan Medical, a division of Kaplan, Inc.
750 Third Avenue
New York, NY 10017

10 9 8 7 6 5 4 3 2 1

Course ISBN: 978-1-5062-5500-2

Retail ISBN: 978-1-5062-5498-2

Kaplan Publishing print books are available at special quantity discounts to use for sales promotions, employee premiums, or educational purposes. For more information or to purchase books, please call the Simon & Schuster special sales department at 866-506-1949.

Editors

Mariana Cuceu, MD

Sherine Elsayegh, MD

Phyllis Levine, MD

Contributor

Edward Kalpas, MD

Curriculum Editor

Ilonka S. Rincon Portas, MD
HEA Associate Director of Facilitation and Clinical Skills
Kaplan Medical

Contributing illustrator: Tejeswini Padma BE, MS

We want to hear what you think. What do you like or not like about the Notes? Please email us at **medfeedback@kaplan.com**.

Table of Contents

Part I: USMLE® Step 2 Clinical Skills Exam

Part II: Communication and Interpersonal Skills (CIS)

Part III: Spoken English Proficiency (SEP)

Part IV: Integrated Clinical Encounter (ICE)

Part V: Putting It All Together

USMLE® Step 2 Clinical Skills Exam

About the USMLE Step 2 Clinical Skills (CS) Exam

The 3-step USMLE examination required for medical licensure in the United States assesses a physician's ability to (a) apply knowledge, concepts, and principles, and (b) demonstrate fundamental patient-centered skills which constitute the basis of safe and effective patient care. Each of the 3 steps complements the others.

Step 1 assesses whether one can understand and apply important concepts of the sciences basic to the practice of medicine. It is based on an integrated content outline which organizes basic science material along 2 dimensions: **system** and **process**. It is a 1-day multiple-choice exam.

Step 2 assesses whether one can apply medical knowledge, skills, and understanding of clinical science essential for the provision of patient care under supervision. It includes emphasis on health promotion and disease prevention. There are 2 components of Step 2.

- **Step 2 CK (Clinical Knowledge)** is based on an integrated content outline that organizes clinical science material along 2 dimensions: physician task and disease category. Step 2 CK uses a 1-day multiple-choice format to test clinical knowledge.

- **Step 2 CS (Clinical Skills)** is a "hands on" exam to test one's ability to gather information from patients, perform physical examinations, and communicate findings to patients and colleagues.

Step 3 assesses whether one can apply medical knowledge and understanding of biomedical and clinical science essential for the unsupervised practice of medicine, with emphasis on patient management in ambulatory settings. It is the final examination in the USMLE sequence.

EXAM OVERVIEW

Step 2 CS is a 1-day live examination which resembles a physician's typical workday in a clinic, doctor's office, ER, and/or hospital setting in the United States. The exam is administered at regional Clinical Skills Evaluation Centers (CSEC) in **Atlanta**, **Chicago, Houston, Philadelphia,** and **Los Angeles**.

- The focus of medical history you need to obtain in each case will be determined by the nature and complexity of the patient's presentation.

- Not every part of the history needs to be taken for every patient. Some patients will have acute problems while others will have more chronic ones.

- You will not have time to do a complete physical exam on every patient, nor is it necessary to do so. Pursue a focused physical examination based on the patient's complaint and information obtained during the history-taking.

Note

The Step 2 CS exam measures skills essential to patient care that cannot be measured by a traditional multiple-choice exam.

Step 2 CS Strategy

It is impossible to do a full physical exam and lengthy patient history in 15 minutes. The key words for this time-critical task are **"pertinent history"** and **"focused physical examination."**

Note

Even though this is a simulated exam, make sure you perform physical examination maneuvers correctly and expect that some encounters may have positive physical findings. Accept any positive findings as real and factor them into your evolving physical diagnoses hypothesis.

The CS exam blueprint is designed to give you a fair representation of cases that a physician is likely to encounter in clinical settings in the United States. Examinees will be required to demonstrate clinical skills most comparable to the level of experience of a first-year medical resident.

Most cases are designed to test the type of history-taking and focused examination that demonstrates your ability to list and pursue plausible differential diagnoses in acute and non-acute situations. Some cases, however, may focus only on history-taking, physical exam, or counseling. Some scenarios, such as phone cases, may involve a parent of a child or a family member of an elderly patient who will not be present in the room. In these situations a physical examination of the patient will not be required; however, you will still be expected to take a history, counsel, articulate a differential diagnosis hypothesis, and write a Patient Note (carefully read the doorway information instructions so you know the tasks that you are expected to perform!).

Clinical case categories include, but are not limited to:

• Cardiovascular	• Neurologic
• Elderly care	• Pediatric care
• Endocrine	• Preventive health
• Gastrointestinal	• Psychiatry
• Genitourinary	• Respiratory
• Musculoskeletal	• Women's health

EXAM SPECIFICS

The exam will include 12 patient encounters. (A very small number of non-scored patient encounters are included for research purposes, but those cases are integrated into the exam.)

- The Evaluation Center where the exam is given will simulate a healthcare environment comparable with a large medical clinic. When you enter the testing area, you will have 12 stations set up as fully equipped examination rooms.
- Each exam room door will post an instruction sheet ("doorway-information"), containing basic information about the case: patient's name, age, gender, reason for the visit, vital signs, and tasks that examinees are expected to perform.
- At the start of each encounter you will hear an announcement such as, *"Examinees you may begin your encounter."*
  - Read the instruction sheet, take notes on the scrap paper, knock on the door, and begin your encounter, just as you would with a real patient. A second copy of the instruction sheet will be accessible in the exam room.
- You will conduct 12 examinations (15 minutes each) of a **"standardized patient"** (SP) chosen from a broad range of age and ethnic backgrounds, and trained to portray a patient with a high degree of reliability.
  - You must communicate with the SPs in a professional and empathetic manner, to establish a good doctor-patient rapport while simultaneously eliciting pertinent historic information and performing a focused physical examination.
  - You must address all the SP's concerns, explain and justify the diagnoses that are being considered, provide counseling when appropriate, inform and get the patient's agreement on planned diagnostic tests.

- After each encounter, you will have 10 minutes to record pertinent history and physical exam findings obtained during the encounter, to list diagnostic impressions (maximum of 3 in the order of likelihood) with support for each, and to outline the diagnostic studies planned.

Step 2 CS at a Glance

Total Exam Length:	8 hours including 2 breaks
Patient Encounters:	12
Length of Each Patient Encounter:	15 minutes
Time Allotted for Writing Each Patient Note:	10 minutes

STRATEGY AND TIME MANAGEMENT

Time management is critical during the CS exam, factoring in the success of your performance.

Patient Encounter: You will be expected to perform **15-minute** patient encounters for **12 SPs** during your exam.

- Each exam room door will have posted the patient's basic information (name, age, presenting complaint, pertinent vital signs, etc.); you must review this information before walking in.
- Assume all doorway information is accurate and use it when generating your differential diagnosis hypothesis.
- Typically, vital signs should not be repeated, but if you do repeat them, refer to the doorway information when developing your differential diagnosis.

Because the exam is standardized, all examinees receive the same information when they ask SPs the same or similar questions. The SPs you encounter during the exam are trained to document your actions in a fair and consistent manner. Immediately following each patient encounter, the SP fills out checklists to document questions you asked, maneuvers you performed, and your demeanor and communication skills including proficiency with the English language during the encounter.

- Based on the patient's presenting complaint, doorway information, and additional information you obtain during the history, consider the most likely possible diagnoses and then explore the relevant ones as time permits.
- To monitor good time management, do the following:
  - During the patient interview, remember that your communication and interpersonal skills are evaluated based on your observable behaviors and your response to the patient's needs.
  - Demonstrate professionalism and good interpersonal/communication skills. Professionalism and public trust go hand-in-hand and they have been viewed as a way to improve patient care and preserve the doctor patient-relationship.
  - Address the patient in a clear manner; your English proficiency is an equally important subcomponent of the CS exam.
  - Demonstrate appropriate clinical skills to obtain a competent history, conduct a focused physical exam, and generate a differential diagnosis and initial work-up using appropriate time management.

Note that certain parts of the physical exam must **not** be done: rectal, pelvic, genitourinary, female breast, corneal reflex, inguinal hernia, and throat swab. If you believe such exams are indicated, include them in the proposed diagnostic workup.

Patient Note: After each encounter, you will have **10 minutes** to record a complete Patient Note that should include:

- All relevant history taken
- Physical examinations performed
- Diagnostic impressions (in order of likelihood) and their supporting data
- Diagnostic workup for initial evaluation

Once you leave the exam room, you are not permitted to re-enter, so be sure you have obtained all necessary information before leaving. However, if you leave the patient encounter early, you can use the additional time to start your Patient Note. In the case of technical or administrative problems, typing the notes on the computer may not be an option. If that happens, you will be required to write your notes by hand. Therefore, be prepared to write one or more Patient Notes on the day of your exam. These notes need to be legible or they cannot be scored.

EXAM COMPONENTS

The CS exam is composed of 3 subcomponents:

- Communication and Interpersonal Skills (CIS)
- Spoken English Proficiency (SEP)
- Integrated Clinical Encounter (ICE)

The **CIS subcomponent** assesses:

- **Fostering the relationship**: listen attentively and show interest, care, concern, and respect
- **Gathering information**: establish chronology of the primary problem, identify patient concerns, and assess impact of health issue on patient
- **Providing information**: explain the most likely diagnosis, encourage and answer questions
- **Helping the patient make decisions**: outline what should happen next linked to a rationale, assess patient's level of agreement and ability to carry out next steps
- **Supporting emotions**: seek clarification of patient's feelings to be sure you are correctly interpreting them, demonstrate understanding, empathy, and support

The **SEP subcomponent** assesses:

- Clarity of spoken English communication within the doctor-patient encounter
- Frequency of pronunciation or word choice errors that affect comprehension
- Listener effort required to understand the examinees questions and responses
- Minimizing the need to repeat questions or statements

The **ICE subcomponent** assesses:

- **Data gathering** skills: patient information collected by history taking and physical examination reflecting your performance during the encounter as well as the documented summary of these findings in your Patient Note
- **Data interpretation** skills: completion of a Patient Note summarizing the findings of the patient encounter, diagnostic impression and justification, and patient diagnostic studies

EXAM SCORING

The Step 2 CS exam is a pass/fail exam. You are scored in each of the 3 subcomponents: ICE, CIS, and SEP. **You must pass all 3 subcomponents on the same day in order to pass.** Failure in one subcomponent will result in failure on the entire exam.

CIS Subcomponent Scoring

Checklists assessing your CIS performance based on observable behaviors are assessed by SPs on all 5 CIS subdivisions:

- Fostering the relationship
- Gathering information
- Providing information
- Helping the patient make decisions
- Supporting emotions

SEP Subcomponent Scoring

Standardized patients (SP) use rating scales to assess the examinees SEP performance.

ICE Subcomponent Scoring

- **Physical Examination checklists** scored by SPs
- **Global ratings** of **Patient Note** scored by trained physicians

A committee of clinicians and medical school clinical faculty develop the checklists.

For your score report, you will receive a Performance Profile covering the strengths and weaknesses of your performance across the 3 subcomponents. The Performance Profile is provided solely for your benefit; it will not be reported to any third parties.

ON TEST DAY

The CS exam begins with an onsite orientation explaining use of the diagnostic equipment available in the exam rooms, test rules, and test procedures. Be sure not to miss this session. At the orientation you will have the opportunity to ask questions.

- The exam lasts about 8 hours, which includes 2 short breaks plus a lunch break.
- A light meal is provided. You may bring your own food, provided that no refrigeration or preparation is required.
- There are vending machines for drinks.

We strongly encourage you to review the orientation video in advance available on the USMLE website. In addition, we recommend the following:

- Arrive at the test center 30 minutes before the scheduled exam.

- Bring your Scheduling Permit and the Confirmation notice.

- An unexpired government-issued form of identification (driver's license or passport) that also has your signature. If the names printed on the 2 documents are different (except for middle names), contact USMLE well ahead of Test Day. Without acceptable level of identification you will not be permitted to take the test.

- Wear comfortable, professional clothing, and a clean white lab or clinic coat.

- Bring an unenhanced standard stethoscope.

- Keep your wallet and driver's license in your pant or coat pocket at all times.

OTHER POINTS TO NOTE

- Wearing a watch is prohibited during the CS exam; a clock is on the wall inside of each patient room, enabling you to follow your time.

- Each exam center contains a locked storage area with small cubicles for storage of necessary personal items; you will be restricted from that area for the entire exam, including breaks.

- Once the on-site orientation has started, you may not leave that area until the exam is over.

- You may not discuss the cases with your fellow examinees at any time.

- Conversation among examinees and with patients in any language other than English is prohibited at all times.

- Proctors will monitor all examinee activity.

- On the day of the exam, you may be asked to sign documents intended to confirm your understanding and willingness to abide by USMLE policies and procedures. You may also be asked to complete demographic and feedback surveys after the exam.

PART II

Communication and Interpersonal Skills (CIS)

Communication and Interpersonal Skills (CIS)

2

The patient–physician relationship should be the center of all clinical medicine. A good relationship starts with good communication skills on the part of the physician. It has been shown to improve patient outcomes, patient satisfaction, as well as physician satisfaction. Contrary to a belief by some physicians, good communication does not prolong an encounter. It can be learned if sufficient time is dedicated to practice and getting feedback.

Effective communication on the exam will allow you to efficiently obtain the information needed during the brief encounter. Expect the standardized patients (SPs) to respond in a realistic way within the confines of their behavioral profiles. The type of responses you receive will sometimes depend on your own personality and characteristics. Following the cooperative responses of the patient, you can determine which body systems to focus on during the physical exam (PE). The patient will become less anxious and more compliant with your requests when you give clear instructions, explain what you are doing each step of the way, and assure the patient that each maneuver is medically important.

Likewise, in closing the encounter, summarize your findings from the history, confirming their accuracy with the patient. Pertinent findings from the PE might be mentioned in the summary as well. Answering any questions the patient may have also gives you a final opportunity to reinforce your competency. Finally, armed with adequate positive and negative findings from the history and physical, you will be able to produce the Patient Note more quickly, with better organization, and with greater accuracy.

The communication skills, along with the PE, are scored by an SP who checks off items on a computerized list as soon as you leave the room. The CIS score is an *average* of the 12 scored encounters; therefore, you could perform awkwardly or ineffectively in 1 or 2 encounters yet still succeed on the exam.

Using the interpersonal skills checklist, the SP rates your skills in interviewing and collecting information, counseling and delivering information, establishing rapport, and maintaining a positive personal manner. Each skill area involves a handful of key characteristics that are important for effective communication in general. Mastery in each area can be achieved by plenty of practice. To deepen and expand self-awareness, seek feedback from the role-playing patient regarding his perception of your interpersonal skills.

TIMING THE PATIENT ENCOUNTER

Time management on the Step 2 CS is crucial. For encounters that require both a history and physical examination, we recommend that you spend up to 1 minute outside the room reviewing the doorway information. Spend 6–7 minutes greeting the patient, eliciting the chief complaint, history of present illness (HPI), and relevant past medical history (PMH), asking about any visible physical findings and related review of systems. Spend 15–30 seconds hand-washing, and then take 3-4 minutes to perform a focused physical exam. Finally, take 3-4 minutes to explain to the patient your findings, counsel, address concerns, and answer any questions.

Note

For each encounter on the exam, you will get a warning that only 5 minutes remain. You should be in the middle of performing the PE when you get this announcement.

Note

A wall clock is present in each room; you may want to write the time of entry so you can keep track of the critical time points noted in the table. Pacing yourself is very important for a higher test score.

1 min	• Read doorway information; copies are in the room and adjacent to the desk where you write the note. • Start thinking of a differential diagnosis list, and write down several of the most likely ones. Jot down a mnemonic if needed. • Knock and enter patient room.
At 7 1/2 min	• End interview (critical point) including writing down key points. This written information will ensure accurate and thorough notes.
From 7 1/2–8 min	• Wash hands and start examination. • Continue the history-taking during the PE.
At 11 1/2 min	• End PE and if needed, write down key points. This written information will ensure accurate and thorough notes.
From 11 1/2–15 min	• Do closing including counseling and end the visit.
From 15–25 min	• Write note.

EVALUATION OF CIS

The following pages present a detailed description of the evaluation of interpersonal and communication skills.

1. Knocked before entering

Knock before going into the examining room. By knocking first, you alert the patient that someone is about to enter. Knocking is a first step in building trust and showing respect. Knock 3 times, wait 3 seconds, open the door and then enter the room. Do not be timid. Even if you are unsure that you heard the SP say "come in," enter after 3 seconds. Do not hesitate and waste valuable time.

> Credit will always be given if you knock. In some cases the SP has been trained to NOT respond to the knock, to see if you will enter or just keep knocking (factors which will affect your use of time and also the relationship).

2. Introduction—used last name and title

Set a tone of friendliness by making a cordial introduction. You will be given credit for introducing yourself by name, greeting the patient by name, and identifying your role in the hospital.

- Introduce yourself using title, first and last name, or title and last name alone. Choose either Dr. Susan Smith or Dr. Smith.
- Do not ever refer to yourself or a patient using first name only.
- Be aware of your word choice throughout the interview. You don't want to sound too informal, and it may even seem unprofessional. At the same time, you don't want to be too formal.
  - If there is any ambiguity in your role, such as your status as a student, explain your relation to the patient's care. If appropriate, you can refer to yourself as a senior medical student or resident on service.

- Many patients will be comfortable receiving a handshake upon introduction. Shake hands if you feel comfortable doing so. A welcoming handshake can serve to relax an anxious patient.
  - However, this form of greeting may not always be appropriate. If a patient is in discomfort, distress, or severe pain, offering a handshake during introduction may not be appropriate. Instead, focus on the patient's comfort by offering to help him move to a more comfortable position.

> Establish eye contact with the SP before you introduce yourself. If you do extend your hand and he does not take it, do not force him to shake. Just withdraw your hand and continue your introduction. Always take your cue from the SP. It shows how well you are focused and paying attention.

3. Established patient's preferred title

Address all patients as "Mr," or "Ms," or "Dr" if they have an advanced degree such as an MD, a DDS or PhD. Then confirm that this is their preferred title.

- Do not use first names only unless the patient requests that you do so. Referring to a patient using a level of formality lower than the level used to refer to yourself would place the patient in an unequal and inferior position.
  - The exception would be a case of an adolescent or child; in that case it is acceptable to use a first name. If you are unsure about the pronunciation of your patient's name, always confirm that you pronounced it correctly.

> Ask the SP what she would prefer to be called or how to pronounce her name if needed. Make sure to use her name periodically throughout the encounter.

4. Clarified role

Explain to the patient your role and your understanding of why the patient has come to be seen by a doctor. This statement informs the patient what will be occurring during the 15-minute encounter.

- For example, "Hello Mr/Ms Jones. I'm Dr. Smith, the clinic or emergency room physician assigned to your care today. I understand you have come here because you xxxxxx (could have pain, are returning for follow-up or annual check-up, want to get test results, are trying to determine if your treatment is working). I will be asking you some questions and examining you, and then discussing my findings and impressions with you."

It is also helpful to align the patient and your expectations about the encounter.

- For example, "Is that your expectation as well?" or "Is that correct?"

This is also a good opportunity to acknowledge that you will be taking notes on important details of the history and physical exam. This will ensure accurate recording of all pertinent information and will help in writing a good Patient Note.

To help establish rapport, start the interaction by asking how the patient is doing today.

- For example, "How are you feeling right now?" If the patient previously had a change in the treatment plan (started a new medication, started on a diet), you can add that to your inquiry. "How have you been doing since you started on x?"

5. Had professional appearance in dress, grooming, and hygiene

A physician's appearance can influence the success of an interview. Patients have an image of what they expect regarding the appearance of a clinician. If you meet those expectations it will build confidence in your medical abilities. Patients form their first impression of you based on your appearance as you enter the room.

- Surveys show patients prefer medical personnel to dress in white coats and wear shoes instead of sneakers. Make sure your white coat is clean and neat.

- Wear comfortable, conservative clothing. It is suggested that men wear trousers, a dress shirt, a tie, and dark shoes, while women wear slacks or a skirt, low-heeled and closed-toe shoes, and conservative jewelry.

- Avoid wearing jeans, sneakers, or sandals.

- Pull your hair back away from your face, trim your nails, and use no products with scents (such as hairspray, perfume, or cologne). You would never want to initiate any allergic reaction in your SP.

- Make sure there are no body or mouth odors or stale clothing odors.

Professional appearance shows that you take pride in yourself, which instills the SP's confidence in you.

---

6. Showed care and concern for patient

- It is important to create an impression that you truly care about the patient. Your overall goal must be to put the patient at ease and diminish the level of anxiety present at the onset of the encounter. This can be accomplished with both verbal and non-verbal (body language).

- Besides choosing appropriate words and phrases, attempt to use a facial expression, posture, and tone of voice that conveys the same message of concern.
    - Look directly at the patient (especially when patient is talking).
    - Avoid writing voluminous notes while conversing.
    - Do not stand during the interview/discussion, because it can make the patient feel that you are controlling, not partnering.
    - Keep an appropriate distance from the patient so you are not too close but also are not across the room.
    - Make sure to appropriately respond to what your patient is saying. If he is talking about losing a job or loved one, sharing that he is in pain, acknowledge your concern and empathy with a statement such as, "I'm so sorry" or "That must be very difficult."

- Patients should leave feeling they had a physician who cared. Typically, patient satisfaction is positively impacted more by a caring, concerned physician that created a welcoming atmosphere than by medical competence.

- Poor positioning may be a sign of discomfort. Ask the patient, "What can I do to make you more comfortable?"
    - If you notice the patient is displaying a negative emotion such as sitting with slumped shoulders and a sad face, acknowledge that you have noticed and are concerned. Say, "I am concerned that something is bothering you. I can't help but notice you look unhappy. Is there something you would like to share with me?" and "I know it may be difficult to open up to a doctor you just met, but I want to help you in any way I can."

- Talking with the patient during the physical exam will reduce her anxiety and increase cooperation. Tell her what you are going to do (e.g., examine the ears), and at times, why (e.g., to look for redness). Proceeding through the physical exam without speaking to the patient will create unnecessary tension and there will be a loss of credit. Maintain eye contact while you are examining the patient so you can determine if anything you are doing is causing her pain or embarrassment.

- You may ask additional questions while performing the physical exam if you are able to maintain eye contact while doing so. However, be careful.

  - For example, asking patients if they have ever had heart trouble when you have just finished listening to the heart, or asking about a family history of cancer after completing a lung exam, may sound scary. Instead, state at the beginning of the physical exam, "As I examine parts of your body, I may ask you some standard questions related to that area. Please do not think that I have found something wrong."

- During the physical exam, be careful of facial expressions or gestures such as a frown that may communicate something is wrong. Patients will often be watching your face for information. A caring expression and tone of voice go a long way to put patients at ease.

- Never alarm patients unnecessarily. When asking certain questions such as "Have you ever been tested for HIV/AIDS?," mention that these questions are routine. Without sufficient information and confirmation, never suggest a catastrophic diagnosis as part of your conclusion.

- Be careful of how you ask a question but also of *when* it is asked. Confronting a difficult subject such as domestic violence too early in an encounter can be inappropriate. Timing is everything.

  - Finding a late point in the history has the advantage of giving you time to establish rapport with the patient and showing your skills at expressing empathy and reassurance. In order to be comfortable enough to open up to you on this difficult subject, patients must truly believe you understand and care.

- Washing your hands in the exam room is another way to show you are concerned about a patient's health. Your cleanliness will protect them from any infectious disease process that could be transmitted from another patient.

  - You will also be given credit if you choose to use gloves. However, wearing gloves creates an unnecessary barrier between you and the patient; therefore, consider using hand washing as your first choice. Resort to gloves only if you have a lesion on your own hands that you do not want to transmit to the patient. If so, be sure to verbalize your reason for this decision.

As you work through the PE, the SP will always feel more comfortable when you talk, letting her know what you plan to do. It's startling to be touched without warning, even if it's a gesture of empathy.

- For example, on a past CS exam an SP played a patient who couldn't open her eyes because of light sensitivity. The doctor touched the patient's hand to reassure her, but he didn't let her know in advance. As a result, the SP was startled and afraid. Had the doctor given a warning, the SP would have perceived that gesture of empathy in a positive way.

---

7. Displayed confident manner and rapport

Always project an image of both confidence and competence throughout the encounter. Patients should feel that you are comfortable in your role as a physician in charge. Things which reflect a lack of confidence include unnecessary pauses during the history or physical examination and repetitively asking, "Is that okay?" Also, talking very fast, tapping your foot, or saying "ummm" can make you appear nervous or insecure.

You are expected to interact with an SP as you would with any real patient, i.e., demonstrate purposeful exploration of relevant components of both the history and physical exam. You will not have time to do a complete physical examination on every patient, only a targeted one. Perform the exam with confidence, being aware and attentive to patient discomfort and modesty. Avoid appearing timid, tentative, unsure, or awkward, and demonstrate a gentle nature.

Remember that the SPs are well trained to mimic the chosen illnesses. This training includes exposure to a very detailed description of the relevant history and physical examination required for each individual case. So in order to appear competent, you must ask the correct types of questions and select the appropriate components of the physical examination.

8. Had respectful and nonjudgmental attitude

Passing judgment on the patient may result in your being considered an unsuitable listener. It is not your role to judge on any patient behaviors such as the use of alcohol and illicit drugs. Your job is to gather the data that will help you make a correct assessment. Showing sensitivity does not mean that you approve of the behavior. If the patient appears uncomfortable, recognize her discomfort and normalize it. "I know discussing these issues can be uncomfortable; however, it is important to know this information for every patient. Is there something I can do to help you feel more comfortable?"

Judgment can be reflected in your choice of words, body language, and even the tone of your voice. Don't ask questions in the negative, such as, "You don't use drugs, do you?" Don't look shocked or surprised if you hear a disturbing answer, and don't raise your eyebrows or frown. Reactions that portray disgust or disapproval will block communication. Be sensitive to all the messages you are sending and control them as best you can. Make sure your facial expression remains consistently respectful.

- It is not necessary to respond after every answer.
- Avoid antagonistic phrases like "You do or did what?" which imply judgment, especially when the question concerns the patient's lifestyle.
- A simple "thank you" or "okay" is often sufficient when the patient is giving information. These responses establish an open, safe atmosphere.
- Reserve all patient education for the end of the encounter.
- Never contradict or impose your standards on the patient. As a rule patients like to respond to questions in a way that attempts to satisfy the physician in order to gain approval. If they perceive that a certain type of answer consistently meets with your approval and another type does not, they may stop providing honest answers to your questions.

Don't move or touch underwear, bras or even gowns, unless requested to do so by the patient, and never touch without explaining first. This applies to draping the patient, untying the hospital gown, and doing anything on the physical examination. Explain what you are doing during every stage of the examination with statements such as "I am going to press on your knee" or "I need to listen to your chest."

> Stay and respond in a neutral manner. If the SP senses judgment, she may not answer your questions truthfully for fear of judgment.

9. Focused attention and concentration on patient

The best way to stay calm under pressure is to focus your attention solely on the patient, and not let yourself be distracted by anything connected to yourself. During the entire 15 minutes you spend with the SP, all you should be doing is establishing a rapport, obtaining sufficient information to generate a diagnostic hypothesis, and considering a plan for how to validate it. Pay close attention to everything the patient says and does. Everything is there for a reason.

During the Step 2 CS exam, take every bit of evidence as a clue. A bandaged wrist may suggest intimate partner violence; a bruise on the upper arm of an elderly patient may indicate elder abuse or a recent fall. If a patient coughs into a handkerchief, ask to see the sputum; hemoptysis may be noted. Remember, the SP will not usually volunteer the very piece of information that could guide your clinical reasoning in a new direction. You will need to be a careful observer. Ask open-ended questions so you don't get a limited answer and miss information. For example:

- Asking if the patient has ever been hospitalized does not mean you are asking if the patient ever had surgery. Surgery can be outpatient and the patient may not assume this is a hospitalization.

- Asking if the patient has any allergies may not reveal a food or seasonal allergy; he may think you only mean an allergy to medications.

- Asking if the patient is on any medication; he may not relay over-the-counter medications because they were not prescribed.

Watch for indications of discomfort from body language such as poor positioning or evidence of pain. Improving the position of the patient may impact your data gathering score. If the patient is more comfortable it will be easier to elicit a good history in a timely fashion. Continue to consider the patient's comfort during the course of the interview. You can make your patient more comfortable by raising or lowering the back of the examining table as needed, by extending the leg rest, or by helping a change in position.

It is key to look at patients when asking questions, giving them your full attention. This will give the impression that you care about them and what is going on with them. In any performance situation, it's possible to become extremely self-conscious and lose focus on the patient. If you become distracted and miss what the patient says, you can say "I'm sorry, could you repeat that? I'm not sure I got it."

Several things may indicate that your attention has wandered from the patient. You may lose points if your eyes wander as you think of your next several questions, if you proceed too slowly or quickly, or if you constantly look at the clock. Do not spend too much time on the clipboard taking notes in excess of that which is necessary. And never leave the patient unnecessarily exposed. To auscultate the heart, for instance, do not raise the gown up from the waist and expose the entire torso; lower the gown instead from the top, exposing only the upper chest and shoulders.

Finally, never assume that anything is so obvious that it does not need to be acknowledged. Any makeup that is used must always be acknowledged. The SP may use appropriate colors to represent trauma, infection, jaundice, or anemia. If you do not verbalize your findings it is as if you did not see what is present and you will lose points on this skill.

> An SP will never try to trick you; everything he does is for a reason. Pay attention and he will guide you through the encounter.
>
> - For example if an SP is wearing socks and all of your other patients were barefoot, there is a reason; find out why. If you need to untie the SP's gown, be sure to retie it before moving on. Make your patient's comfort your priority.

10. Listened attentively without interrupting

If a patient doesn't immediately answer a question you have asked, wait in silence for patients to think about the answers to your questions and sometimes to process their feelings. Once speaking, patients' answers should not be cut off. Let them finish speaking, even if there are pauses and silences. Interrupting disrupts their train of thought. Quietly wait for each answer to be completed and don't fill in words for the patient. Grant them the proper respect of being heard fully. If the question has hit on a sensitive issue and the patient becomes teary, offer a tissue, sit down, and quietly wait. In general, a brief pause or silence will encourage patients to say more. Silence is one of the least invasive interviewing techniques, one that encourages the patient to open up and share more freely. However, if the silence becomes prolonged, observe for signs of distress since a prolonged silence may be indicative of distress. You can address this by recognizing the patient's distress and your role in causing it. You could state, "You seem distressed and I'm so sorry that my questions have upset you. This information is important, so is there anything I can do to assist you or should we come back to this a little later?"

Don't worry about the lack of time in a sensitive case like grieving or depression; never lose sight of the human connection. The Step 2 CS exam is primarily a test of interpersonal and communication skills. Step 2 CS cases are carefully planned to take approximately 15 minutes, including any expression of emotion or hesitation on the part of the SP.

Of course, at times, it may be necessary to interrupt patients. They may be talking on and on about irrelevant matters, such as a problem a family member may be having. In such cases, you can gain the patients' trust even more strongly by firmly interrupting to refocus on them. Cut in whenever patients hesitate slightly, look them straight in the eyes, and say, "Excuse me for interrupting, Ms. Jones." Next, acknowledge whatever the patient was talking about by stating, "I know these concerns have really been troubling you, and we can discuss them at a follow-up visit." Then bring the focus back to the patient: "However, right now I want to focus completely on you." Chances are they will feel validated that someone cares enough to want to focus on their symptoms.

Avoid repeating the same question, unless for clarification. If you are unsure what a patient has said or think an answer is vague, ask the question again, explaining that you are trying to verify that you heard correctly. Sometimes patients will answer the same question using different words and therefore the meaning will be clearer.

Occasionally there may be an inconsistency between a fact stated later in the history compared to an earlier stated fact. Therefore, you may need to ask for clarification to be sure you have obtained the correct information.

Never quickly repeat a question before the SP has had time to respond. It may appear that you don't care whether the response is accurate—just that it is given rapidly.

> Learn to feel comfortable with silence. When you give the SP time to think and respond, she feels respected and heard. SPs are very aware of 15 minutes; they have been trained to think and to hesitate in responding to see if you will interrupt. At the same time, however, they will not impede you from completing your encounter in the allotted 15 minutes. An SP may speed up or shorten responses, but she will always include all the information you asked for as long as she is not interrupted.

11. Maintained comfortable eye contact

Position yourself so that the patient can easily see you without straining. Attempt to maintain your eyes as close as possible to being at the same level as those of the patient. If the patient is lying down facing either right or left, move around to that side of the table and sit down at a slight angle so that patients do not need to extend their necks. Sitting down is considered a positive behavior by American patients because it projects time to listen and concentrate.

When you encounter patients lying on their backs, remember to stand but also at a slight angle.

Patients should not have to turn their heads to see you. Never stand behind the patient during the history or the closing. If the patient is sitting at the end of the table, sitting down would be less intimidating and would help create a better initial rapport between you and the patient.

In general, if you seem to be avoiding eye contact or look distracted, you will not be seen as listening to or caring about the patient. Comfortable eye contact reinforces a sense of trust and credibility. If you shift your eyes around the room or avoid looking directly at the patient, you may communicate a lack of self-confidence.

Even during physical examination eye contact remains important. For example, you may need to observe the patient's face for any signs of pain or discomfort.

> Staring at the SP will make him feel awkward and uncomfortable. He would prefer you to look and listen with interest and concern, without staring into his eyes or at a specific body part.

12. Maintained comfortable and appropriate distance

Standing too close or too far away may suggest either a stance of aggression or timidity, respectively. As a general rule, 2 feet is about right for personal proximity in the American culture. Observe for cues from the SP. If the patient continuously leans back, you are probably too close. If the patient leans forward, you are probably too far. It is appropriate to stand closer to a patient suffering from bilateral hearing loss.

13. Used proper draping technique

Many patients will already be covered to the waist with the drape. If not already on the patient, the drape sheet may be folded on the stool in the examining room. Before you begin the medical interview, reach for the drape, unfold it halfway, and place it immediately on the patient from the waist down. Before covering the patient, say "I'd like to cover you now to make you feel a little more comfortable." That way, you are indirectly asking for permission and showing empathy for the patient's comfort. You can also encourage the patient to adjust the drape to maximize his own comfort.

- Strictly speaking, as long as you drape the patient no later than the beginning of the physical exam, you should receive credit. However, it is preferable to do so at the beginning of the history since the drape is on the stool upon which you will be sitting. It makes logical sense to do it first since you won't want to sit on the drape you will be using later.
- The one exception to this general rule is that any patient lying down must be draped even before beginning the history.

As soon as you have completed examining a particular section of the body, replace the drape without delay. Also, if part of the examination involves asking the patient to stand, replace the drape after the patient returns to the table.

Regarding the hospital gown, prior to beginning the physical examination, create a mutually agreed upon plan with the patient. Some patients will prefer to have the physician untie, retie, raise, and lower the gown; some will prefer to do those things themselves; some will prefer to share the hospital gown responsibilities. Whatever decision is made will hold for the entire physical exam and the issue will not have to be discussed again during each portion of the exam.

> The drape is not just for covering your SP; it gives you the opportunity to really see your patient. You are covering him and focusing on him. Observe his physical, mental, and emotional demeanor. This moment may tell you more than the doorway scenario.

14. Non-verbal communication

There are various ways to show patients that, as their physician, you are focused on what they are saying and want to hear more.

- Nod your head
- Lean in toward the patient
- Use sufficient short pauses and at times, use long appropriate silences
- Maintain an engaged listening posture
- Do not cross your arms or place your hands in your pockets

15. Elicited chief complaint (CC)

One method is to begin the history with an open-ended question such as, "What caused you to come see me today?" An alternative approach would be to repeat the chief complaint stated in the doorway information and then verify that it is the chief complaint.

- "My nurse told me you came here today for [CC]. Is that correct?
- "I would like to hear in your own words what has been bothering you."

For most cases the CC stated in the doorway information will be the same complaint stated by the patient in the room. However, on occasion, the patient may have not been comfortable telling the intake person the actual complaint since it may have felt too private. That patient may have found it difficult to disclose the real complaint to anyone besides the physician. For these cases, the patient may change the CC from the one stated on the door.

- A 60-year-old man suffering from erectile dysfunction may initially state to the nurse an unrelated urinary or gastrointestinal complaint, but then tell the physician about his sexual dysfunction.

16. Established timeline of chief complaint (CC)

The patient must feel that the physician is attempting to elicit as much background information as possible regarding the chief complaint and to understand what may be causing it to occur. The SP will not necessarily be looking for specific questions but rather for the presence of a thought process that uses characteristics of the complaint as well as other associated symptoms and their timing in relation to the chief complaint. The physician is not being graded on a specific history checklist as part of data gathering but rather on an overall impression created on the SP that reflects the ability to do a logical targeted history.

17. Asked open-ended questions

Open-ended questions are those that require a sentence or two describing something in the patient's own words and encourage a longer, more detailed response. They do not limit the response the patient can provide. Begin with general open ended questions to enable patients to tell you as much as they want about the current problem. For example "What caused you to come see me today?" This allows them to begin with their own narrative. Then proceed to more directed open-ended ones to help focus the questioning. For example, "What makes your pain worse?"

You can also end your history with one last open-ended question such as "Is there anything else you would like to tell me about your health that we did not discuss?"

> When you do not use open-ended questions, the SP does not feel encouraged to tell her story. She will merely answer yes or no without any detail.

18. Followed up with close-ended questions

Close-ended questions will be answered with a simple yes/no or a few words. Close-ended questions will fill in specific details not already provided by the patient. If asked too early, relevant information may be lost. For example, if your case is about a patient with lower abdominal pain, you should have in mind some associated symptoms by the time the initial history questions have been answered. Asking "Do you have diarrhea?" or "Have you been feeling nauseated?" will yield a more direct answer than "Do you have any other symptoms?" If asked that way the SP would probably say, "Like what?" Typically at the end of the history of present illness, closed ended questions will help you identify patterns of symptoms characteristic of the common diseases tested on the CS exam. In addition, most questions regarding past medical history will be asked as closed-ended ones.

A fine balance can be struck between these two types of questioning. Proceed from the more general to the more specific ones. That way, patients will initially be able to express what is important to them and you will still be able to obtain detailed, significant, and accurate data in a timely fashion.

> Asking about "change"—any change in sleep, diet, bowel habits, etc.—saves time and lets the SP tell the story. Closed-ended questions should logically follow from open-ended questions (thus, use no non-sequitors). When done this way, the SP will find it easy to follow your line of questioning.

19. Used non-leading questions

Questions should be stated in a neutral manner to avoid leading the patient into answering in a way that compromises accuracy. Neutrality is achieved by using the affirmative mode, rather than the negative: "Mr. Brown, have you ever used tobacco products?" instead of "You don't smoke, do you?" "Any nausea or vomiting?" instead of "No nausea or vomiting?" Questions should be asked in a way that encourages patients to answer candidly without fear of being judged or blamed for behaviors that can compromise their health, such as smoking cigarettes. If you were to say to a patient "You don't smoke, do you?" the patient might be uneasy about revealing the true history.

Be careful about leading your patients down a path framed from your own assumptions. For example, ask a patient with vaginal bleeding and clots "What did the clot look like?" rather than "Did the clot look like a piece of liver?" Your concept of a piece of liver may be based primarily on size while that of the patient may be based on texture. In other words, you may be asking if it was a large smooth clot, while the patient who responds yes may be telling you just that the blood looked smooth. If allowed to describe the clot to you, the same patient may say "It looked like a grape" which would reflect a much smaller clot.

20. Asked clear and concise questions

It is important to ask only one question at a time. Ask the question, then pause and wait for an answer before going on to the next one. Don't barrage the patient with a string of questions. Too often physicians run questions together in a list. "Has anyone in your family ever had high blood pressure, high cholesterol, strokes, or any heart condition that you know of?" "Have you had any nausea, vomiting, constipation or diarrhea?" Separate these items and ask them one at a time. Otherwise, the patient will become confused and feel rushed. Out of a sense of sheer confusion the patient may simply say no.

In addition, you will have used poor time management by running questions together in this way. The SP will probably say, "What? Which one?" and then you will have to start all over again. Worse yet, the SP may respond only to the final question in a string of questions, thus misleading you into thinking that the answer applies to all the previous parts as well and thereby undermining your clinical reasoning.

Asking questions without giving the patient an opportunity to answer interferes with clear communication. However, it is acceptable to use a list of questions if the choices are mutually exclusive and there is only one correct choice from the entire list. For example, you can ask your patient "Are your sexual partners male, female, or both?" It is also acceptable to ask simple combination questions of 2 items routinely grouped together such as, "Any nausea or vomiting?" "Any tingling or numbness?" or "Any fever or chills?"

> When asked several questions at a time, the SP has been trained to answer only the last one with a simple "yes" or "no." The result: you may be misled.

21. Paraphrased and checked-in with the patient

All through the encounter, briefly either repeat back or rephrase a patient's key words based on your understanding of the stated facts. Repeating back the last few words of a sentence, echoing, and then pausing, will encourage your patient to give you more details. Interpreting what you just heard will not only show the patient that you are listening but will also provide an opportunity to correct any wrong information.

Shortly after discussing the chief complaint (by having asked, "What caused you to come in today?") and obtaining answers to a few other follow-up questions, it is a good idea to reflect the main points to the patient. Afterward, ask, "Is that correct?" If you've misunderstood any part of the response, the patient can then clarify. Paraphrasing will assist you greatly in your clinical reasoning. You need not repeat back the exact statement of the patient but rather your interpretation that reflects that you understood both the content and meaning of the statement.

Here are some examples of reflection and paraphrasing:

Doctor: "I see you're wearing an Ace bandage on your wrist. What happened there?"

Patient: "Oh, I hurt my wrist playing pool yesterday."

Doctor: (Nodding) "Playing polo?"

Patient: "No, no—playing pool."

Doctor: "Oh, okay. Playing pool."

Doctor: "Have you had any change in your weight lately?"

Patient: "Yeah, I've lost about 7 or 8 pounds."

Doctor: "Over what period of time?"

Patient: "Let's see—over about the past 2 months."

Doctor: "So you were in good health until 2 months ago when you began to lose weight, is that correct?"

Doctor: "Has your weight changed lately?"

Patient: "Yes, I must have lost about 7 or 8 pounds."

Doctor: "Over what length of time?"

Patient: "About 2 months."

Doctor: "So you've lost about 7 or 8 pounds over the past 2 weeks?"

Patient: "No, not 2 weeks; it's been about 2 months."

Doctor: "Oh, 2 months. All right."

Finally, remember that paraphrasing provides you with a good opportunity to take a few notes. Since you initially are not gathering any new information, a break in eye contact will be accepted by the patient.

> When you paraphrase information back to the SP, even if it's just a phrase such as "vomited once, no blood," the SP feels heard. It also gives the SP the opportunity to make sure you are both 'on the same page.

22. Elicited additional, including hidden, concerns

In order for patients to leave the encounter satisfied, all their concerns must be identified and addressed. The patients will not always openly volunteer this information. Many concerns remain hidden and will only come out when a dedicated physician probes for all of them. You must help patients achieve their specific goals in seeking medical care.

Not every patient with the same chief complaint has the same hidden concerns. These concerns result from an individual's unique history and past exposures. One patient with abdominal pain may fear cancer as a result of having a family member with similar pain who was diagnosed with cancer. Another patient may fear surgery as a result of having undergone a prior surgical procedure that resulted in multiple postoperative complications. To address these varying concerns, the physician must be aware of them. Therefore, always ask patients, "What worries you the most about your CC?"

Another category of hidden concerns relate to family history. Many patients fear that they too are either at risk of or in the process of developing the same diseases that plagued other family members. This is especially true if they personally viewed the day to day difficulties the family member experienced or if they were present when that family member succumbed to the disease. Therefore, it is important to also identify these hidden concerns.

> A clue of some kind will usually be given by the SP that there is a hidden concern which should be addressed. This clue could be a verbal comment, a change in tone or speech pattern, an emotional reaction, or a simple shift in physical presence. Stay focused on your patient and you will witness the change in demeanor.

23. Asked about impact on patient's life

Ask directly how the presenting symptom has affected the patient's daily activities, family, or work. The symptom may have impacted the patient in a physical, psychological, or social way. Obviously a more long-standing complaint will have had the opportunity to more significantly impact the life of the patient. However, even a complaint that only began several hours prior to presentation may have already affected the patient. One patient may have been in the process of completing a major work project with a deadline that evening and had to leave work to seek care. Another patient may be a single parent who was at home caring for two small children and could not find anyone to watch them and therefore had to bring these children to the emergency room. Knowing the specific impact on any individual enables the physician to address the concerns and needs specific to that patient.

> No matter how minor the chief complaint, it will have an impact on the life of the patient (even if it's just a matter of the time taken to come to the clinic).

24. Asked what patient thought was going on

Prior to delivering the diagnostic impression, it is recommended to ask the patient, "What do you think is causing your symptom?" Care must be taken to ask this question in the proper context so as not to receive an answer from the patient such as, "Why are you asking me that? You are the physician."

Be sure to explain to the patient the reason for your question.

- "I want to be sure that I address any concerns you may have and correct any misinformation you may have obtained from the media or other sources. I also want to be sure that I provide you with enough information to fully understand the probable cause of your symptom and to meet your expectations of this visit."
  - Attempt to see the presenting complaint through the eyes of the patient and understand the patient's perspective.

> Patients are smart and they have the internet. They will always have an idea of 'what's going on' with them, whether they tell you or not. Ask them what they think.

25. Used lay language or offered explanation

Patients should be regarded as knowing very little about the meaning of specialized medical terminology, so be sure to choose words and phrases that they will easily understand. Use language which any speaker of English can understand, with or without a specialized education. Furthermore, never undermine a positive rapport with the patient by showing off your technical expertise using medical jargon.

Medical jargon can easily creep into conversation. This is especially true if the word seems commonplace to you, such as *trauma, hypertension,* or *CT scan.*

- If you accidentally use a technical or medical term, explain immediately what it means in simple, straightforward language. The SP will give credit on this basis.
  - If you use medical terminology without explaining or if the patient has to ask what a term means, credit will not be given.

When preparing for your CS exam, be sure that you are able to describe in plain language what is going on in the patient's body and what tests you will be ordering. Never assume that patients will understand even simple medical terms such as *hypertension* that have become part of everyday speech.

- Patients may not tell you they don't understand a term you used, and will leave the encounter without being fully informed.

> When you use medical jargon without explaining in simpler terms, the SP may feel inferior and even stupid. She may hesitate to ask for an explanation, which could cause her to leave with incorrect information. If you use medical terms, always clarify what they mean.

26. Incorporated appropriate use of continuers

Many short phrases and statements exist which inform patients that you, as the physician, would like to hear more information on a particular subject. They will typically encourage the patient to continue speaking. Learn to incorporate some of these statements into your clinical encounters.

- "I see"
- "Uh-huh, go on"
- "Mm-hmm"
- "Tell me more"
- "Yes, and then"

27. Incorporated appropriate use of transitions

Transitions (i.e., transitional words and phrases) are like signposts, alerting patients that you have obtained sufficient information on the current subject and are ready to move to a new area of questioning. For example, they will signal that you are moving from the history to the PE, and then to the closing.

- Transitional statements allow patients to follow along with the logic of your inquiry and thus keep the communication clear. By conveying an impression of orderly thinking, transitions will foster confidence and trust in your judgment.
- Increase sensitivity by always including a transition before embarking on the components of the personal social history and reminding and reassuring patients that what they will now tell you will be kept confidential. At this point you can also say to the patient "If you prefer, I will not write down your answers."

- Sometimes also reminding patients that these are routine medical questions asked of most patients will help them discuss something which may be difficult.
- Appropriate places to present a transitional statement are before the past medical and family histories; before the personal social history, i.e., questions about substance abuse including tobacco and alcohol, sexual history, intimate partner violence, and—in some cultures—menses; before the physical exam; moving from one region to another; and closing.

- **Before the past medical history:**

  "Okay, Mr. Green, now I'm going to ask you some questions about your health in general."

- **Before the sexual history:**

  "I am now going to ask you some personal questions regarding your sexual history. The answers will help me determine the reasons for your symptoms. Everything we discuss today will be kept confidential."

- **Before the social history:**

  "Thank you. Now let me ask you about your work and home life."

- **Before asking questions about smoking, alcohol, and recreational drug use:**

  "Okay, now I need to get some information about your habits and lifestyle."

- **Before the family history:**

  "Now let's talk about your family's health."

- **Before the physical exam:**

  "Thanks for answering all these questions. Now I'll need to examine you. Excuse me while I first wash my hands."

- **Before the closing:**

  "Thank you, Mrs. Jones. I have finished with my examination. I'd like to now sit down and discuss what I think so far."

> Without transitions, questions can be abrupt and confusing. Patients prefer to know what is happening next. Keep your SP informed and on track by using transitions.

28. Summarized significant information

Recent studies have shown that there is a strong positive relationship between the time spent doing the closure and the outcome on the CIS component of the CS exam. Therefore, be sure to give yourself enough time at the end of each encounter to complete your closure. This is your opportunity to pull everything together.

Before sharing your diagnostic impression, summarize 4 to 5 important points from the history and physical exam which have led to your preliminary conclusions. These points may be either pertinent positives or pertinent negatives. Remember this is part of your communication score and if you do not report the information accurately it will reflect negatively on your listening skills.

In order to use the limited amount of time provided for each encounter most efficiently, summarize only after completing both your history and physical examination. There is no need to stop and summarize at the completion of the history and then again after completing the physical examination. Your summary will be more complete and informative once all data gathering has been completed.

29. Delivered diagnostic impression

Next you need to state your diagnostic impression to the patient. First give the diagnosis in medical terms and then explain what the diagnosis means. Here, medical terminology should be used combined with an appropriate explanation.

- "I think you most likely have an ectopic pregnancy, which is a pregnancy growing outside of your womb."

Including the actual disease name shows respect for the intellectual capacity of the patient. Also, patients will feel comforted knowing that after the visit they have the ability to investigate on their own and learn more about their possible diagnosis. Once again, information can be comforting to patients. It is better to explain one disease properly than to list other possibilities in an unexplained fashion.

Many times the diagnosis you suspect is the most likely diagnosis for the case is one that is much less serious and more easily resolved than the one told to you by the patient when asked what the patient thinks is the cause of the chief complaint. If so, remember to inform the patient that you do not think they have the concerning disease. If the suspected diagnosis is more severe than suspected by the patient, you must frame the conversation differently and be prepared for a stronger reaction by the patient to the diagnosis.

When explaining the diagnosis to patients, consider referring to an organ or body system (heart, lungs, liver, immune system) and then state the general condition of that organ or system (infection, virus, blockage, inflammation). Remember that this is not a definitive but rather a possible diagnosis.

> When delivering the diagnosis, watch the SP carefully. If you have not yet pursued hidden concerns (item 22), this may be the moment when the SP will react based on his fears and concerns. If you missed this clue, the SP knows you were not focused on him.

30. Justified diagnosis

The SPs are well trained to play these cases and are quite knowledgeable about the mimicked diseases. Therefore, your choice of supporting facts from both the history and physical exam must accurately justify the given probable diagnosis. Also remember that you are being graded on your communications skills, where *how* you say something is relatively more important than what you say. Even if the diagnosis you select is not the most likely diagnosis for the case, but rather an appropriate differential diagnosis, you will still receive credit if it is explained properly and can be justified using the facts of the case.

31. Addressed patient's need for additional information

Illness will always be frightening to patients. Most often they will assume the worst possible cause of their symptoms. One thing that you as their physician can do to alleviate their fear is to help them understand what is happening. By providing patients with sufficient medical information in an understandable format you can put them at ease. Remember that you are trying to *decrease* uncertainty, not increase it, in your patients.

Carefully observe the patient's response to the diagnosis and later on to the proposed required tests. If the patient looks puzzled or says something like "Why do you think that is what is causing my CC or that this test will help confirm what is wrong?" remember to explain in further detail. The amount of information required by different patients may depend on their personality, level of education, or level of distraction by the seriousness of the CC.

> If you acknowledge the SP's reaction to the diagnosis, it will lead you to determine whether he will want additional information. Focus on the SP and he will guide you.

32. Encouraged and answered questions

Always encourage the patient to ask questions—it is better to state, "What questions do you have?" instead of "Do you have any questions?" because the latter can be answered with yes/no. Then answer briefly in a clear and reassuring manner. Typically the SP should ask only the number of questions that can reasonably be answered in the available time. If you are asked more than you are capable of answering in the allotted time, reassure the patient that you will address all concerns at the follow-up visit.

- "I wish I had more time today to answer all your questions and address all your concerns. We can begin our next visit discussing the other issues you mentioned today."

> You have been asking the SP a number of questions for 14 minutes, and now he may want to ask one of you. Ask if he has any questions.

33. Assessed patient's comprehension of probable illness

Once you have provided the patient with all the information you deem necessary to understand the diagnosis, you must confirm with the patient that you have succeeded in achieving this goal. Ask if anything else needs to be clarified. By the time you leave the examining room, the patient should feel adequately informed, supported, and ready to take the next step.

> When the SP is informed and understands his situation, he will feel empowered.

34. Clearly stated next steps

By the end of the encounter, the patient should know what to do next. In most cases, this is accomplished by your stating which tests are necessary. Technical terminology should not be used in specifying lab work; however, it is imperative that you explain the purpose of the test. Never just say that we need to do further investigations with a vague reference to a test.

- "I will order a blood test to see if you have an infection."
- **NOT** "I will order a blood test" (too vague) or "I will order a CBC" (too technical)

This section also presents an additional opportunity to thank patients for sharing all the previously given information and letting them know that the information has helped in selecting the most appropriate tests to clarify their symptoms and confirm the correct diagnosis.

> Patients like to know what to do next. After informing the SP of the tests required, tell her what to do next, such as get dressed or relax in her seat until the nurse or technician comes.

35. Counseled the patient

It is very difficult to get patients to change their habits and lifestyle and to commit to following medical recommendations. It often helps for them to have family and/or friends who would be willing to assist. Therefore, try to identify the support network of your patients prior to introducing counseling. Then one thing you can suggest might be to have the patient involve one of those individuals in the process. Include any support available in the hospital or community, such as counseling or peer support groups for diabetes, lupus, cancer, etc. and social services for any financial concerns. Your goal should be to build a supportive therapeutic relationship with your patient.

Also, patients will more likely comply with your recommendations if they understand why they should do them. Raising their anxiety level a bit without overly alarming them can be effective.

- "As your physician I want you be as healthy as possible, so I am sending you to our counselor at the hospital who can help you cut down on the number of cigarettes you are smoking each day," **ADDING** "since cigarettes can harm your heart and lungs."

Another key point is to present counseling information to patients with empathic understanding about their clinical status. For example, a patient with severe recurrent hemoptysis and a history of cigarette smoking should be provided with plans for the management of the acute problem. Cigarette smoking can be addressed when the patient has improved.

- "A chest x-ray is needed, which I will review immediately. If you wish, I will provide you with information to help you stop smoking. It may be playing a role here, but let's first take care of this immediate problem."

Patients can be counseled about issues related to their general health and disease prevention, such as going for routine medical visits and age appropriate screening tests, diet, exercise, safe sex, cigarette and alcohol cessation, and compliance with prescription medications. Occasionally, counseling can be more specific and related directly to the CC such as not driving with a seizure disorder.

> SPs feel 'taken care of' and confident when you counsel them in a non-judgmental manner. They know you are concerned about their health and best interest; when you treat them as a partner, it will make them more open and compliant with the proposed treatment.

36. Agreed to a mutual plan of action

During the encounter, you as the physician will advise the patient of the necessity to make lifestyle changes which will improve health and well-being. In addition, you will specify the tests needed to definitively diagnose the cause of the presenting complaint. To achieve these goals, the patient must agree to comply with all of your recommendations.

The patient needs to realize that you will always be available to help with this process. Make statements that are suggestive of a plan of action based on mutual involvement. Shared decision-making that includes the participation of the patient will create solutions that best fit the needs and personality of the individual patient.

- "We are a team."
- "We will figure this out together."
- "Let's work on this together."
- "How does this sound to you?"
- "Do you agree with this plan of action?"

Note

You will be given credit for verbal counseling. However, USMLE guidelines clearly state that counseling should be omitted from the Patient Note since it is not considered part of the diagnostic plan.

It is imperative to uncover any barriers that could potentially interfere with achieving your stated goals. The patient must have both the motivation and capability to succeed. If a patient is not ready to agree to all your medical suggestions, the proposed and accepted mutual plan of action may be simply for the patient to agree to come for a follow-up visit and continue the discussion.

37. Actively listened and validated patient's experience

The final step in the process of showing empathy involves validating the patient's emotions. You may not agree with the emotion but you accept it without judgment and respect his right to feel that way. Be sure that patients feel legitimized and leave thinking that you accept them wholeheartedly with both their strengths and weaknesses.

- "Many of my patients with similar problems have felt the way you do."
- "I can understand why you would be worried under these circumstances. It would be surprising if you were not worried."
- "I can image that I would feel as you do if I had been through that."

38. Expressed empathy with appropriate reassurances

Empathy shows that you accurately understand what the patient is feeling and why they are feeling as they do. It starts with demonstrating to the patient that you understand, yet as the physician you are maintaining a level of emotional detachment. Every case should begin and end with an expression of empathy, with additional expression and non-verbal displays of empathy at appropriate times.

There are several types of situations that will give you the opportunity to prove your capacity to express empathy, and therefore be given exam credit for verbal expression of empathy.

- Patients describe emotions they are currently feeling, whether very positive or very negative about something physical or psychosocial
- Patients are open and tell you directly their concerns and how feeling this way has impacted their lives
- Patients simply state how they feel and need you to probe for additional details ("What do you think brought this on?" or "Tell me how this has affected you?")
- Patients simply state how they feel such as "my stomach really hurts," "I am so tired all the time," or "lately I don't seem to be able to concentrate on my job."
  - In these cases, acknowledge the statement and then ask about concerns connected to that statement. One patient with abdominal pain may fear she has cancer, another may be worried about the possible need for surgery, and yet another may worry that if it is something contagious she will not have anyone to take care of her children. You must determine the implications of that complaint to your individual patient.

Besides asking about the patient's concerns, as an alternative approach you can suggest how you think this problem has affected the patient. Do not merely acknowledge the complaint but explain what you think having the chief complaint means to the patient and how it may have affected them. If a patient presents with severe knee pain, show that it is important to you to understand the effect the pain has had on the patient's quality of life.

- "I can see you are in a lot of pain" ADDING "It must be difficult for you to walk around and perform many of your daily tasks."

Either way, by inviting further discussion on the subject and giving patients a chance to elaborate further, you are showing them that you are both listening and want to truly understand their feelings. Your patient should feel listened to as well as understood. Avoid statements such as "I know how you feel" or "I know what you are going through" because that may be considered presumptuous, trite, robotic, generic, or insincere. You never want the patient to feel that you shifted the focus from them to you.

The final step in this process of showing empathy involves receiving confirmation from patients that you as the physician truly understood what they were feeling and why they feel that way. That confirmation will come in statements such as "Thank you for listening. That is exactly how I feel." or "Wow. You really understand how I am feeling." or simply "Yep. You got it."

The second type of situation that will give you an opportunity to express empathy will be more observational in nature. Learn to notice and interpret the nonverbal cues of patients who are anxious, sad, or angry.

- Patients are sitting with shoulders slumped, a sad facial expression, sighing and holding their bodies tensely, or breaking eye contact

    - In these cases, comment on what you notice and ask if there is something the patient would like to share verbally with you connected to their non-verbal communication. Even silence may indicate that the patient is feeling something deeply and trying to control emotions.

    - On your part, empathic expression also involves non-verbal communication. Verbal and nonverbal communication should complement each other. Empathy can be communicated through facial expressions, appropriate body posture, mannerisms, and tone of voice. Changing your tone of voice can change the entire meaning of your words and can be used to acknowledge the patient's feelings and to show a genuine desire to help.

Sometimes a simple gesture like an appropriate placement of a hand on a patient's shoulder communicates warmth, caring, and support. Assisting a patient to lie down or sit up by holding an arm or back demonstrates that you understand that it may be difficult to do so without help. Even a simple nod, or leaning in to listen, conveys to the patient that you are listening, absorbing information, and trying to understand.

Finally, while performing the PE, exhibiting appropriate caution can convey to patients an understanding of their current circumstances. Always examine the asymptomatic areas prior to the symptomatic ones. Warn the patient in advance prior to doing something unexpected or painful. If the patient appears to be in significant pain, when inquiring about the hospital gown, remembering to verbalize that you recognize that any shifting of position required to move the gown may exacerbate the pain, once again conveys understanding.

Be attentive to patient discomfort and do not cause any unnecessary pain by performing any maneuvers that yield no new data. If you suspect appendicitis and the psoas test is positive, do not perform an obturator test. Similarly, do not ask the patient to change positions more often than necessary, which could cause unnecessary pain. (This could happen if, to complete your evaluation, you wanted to return to an area previously examined and thus asked a patient in pain to change position once again.)

The best way to communicate that you truly understand will be with appropriate reassurance. Be sure that your reassurances are consistent with the expectations and concerns of the patient.

- It is inappropriate to assure patients that they will get well or be cured, or to say that the condition isn't serious and not to worry if it is not. Reassure them instead that you will be extremely thorough and will help them get through this difficult time.

- Emphasize to patients that they are in a safe, modern medical center with an excellent medical staff.

- Offer your personal support and let patients know they are not alone.

Do not provide false reassurances with statements such as, "Don't worry, everything is going to be fine." Trust will not develop if the discussion is dishonest. If the patient is worried about something, she should be encouraged to speak further. Otherwise patients may think you do not take their feelings seriously.

It is important that you find empathic phrases which feel natural to you.

- That sounds very frustrating.
- This must be very frustrating for you.
- I notice that you seem to be feeling xxx.
- I want to understand what happened.
- I want to understand your feelings.
- What you seem to be saying is…is that correct?
- Can I help you put your feelings in words.
- Some people feel…. how do you feel?
- Am I hearing you right?
- It must be very difficult for you to cope with this.
- I recognize that this is a difficult time for you.
- I can understand how that could be upsetting.
- It sounds like you have been through a lot lately. I can understand how you would be upset.
- Let me make sure I understand your concerns.
- You seem angry, sad, etc.
- You seem to be having trouble telling me about….
- It must be terrible feeling tired all the time where everything takes so much effort. Tell me how it affects you.
- What do you think might be going on?
- What do you think brought this on?
- How does that affect you?
- What do you fear most about this?

> Observe the SP and then acknowledge what you see in a sincere non-robotic way. Don't say you "know how he feels" since you may never have had the same experience. Acknowledge what you see—the mental, emotional, or physical state—and then offer reassurance that you are here for support.

39. Inquired about patient's support system

Patients will require help and support to deal with both acute and chronic problems. Support can include family, friends, work colleagues, clergy, therapists, support groups, and financial counselors. The form of support needed will depend on the situation. A patient who has to remain in the hospital may need emotional support as well as help with home and work obligations that cannot be fulfilled during the hospitalization. A person who needs to introduce lifestyle modifications such as an exercise regimen or a new diet may need a companion who has sufficient time available to eat and exercise with the patient.

Begin by asking the patient who in his life is available for support, and then offer additional and alternative support as needed. Most importantly, be sure that the patient knows you are always available to help in any way you can. Your recognition of the difficulty of achieving certain goals without appropriate support, as well as your commitment to help, reinforces the partnership you have created with the patient during the encounter.

40. Managed the challenge

Most challenges are testing one of several possible things. The first may be your ability to recognize an emotion the patient is displaying and why they may be feeling that way. If you encounter an angry patient, try to figure out why he is angry. He may state that he is angry because you made him wait so long to see you, but his anger might be indicative of something deeper and more complicated. In other words, his anger may be displaced; perhaps he is afraid of something such as being seriously ill for this first time or of losing control in a medical setting. Accept the fact that the patient is angry and do not get angry in return. Maintain your level of professionalism and composure and never become defensive.

Other challenges will be created to see if you, as a physician, are secure enough to admit further information is needed before you can commit to a diagnosis or treatment. Examples may be challenges from patients asking "Do I have cancer?" or "Am I going to die?" Be sure to explore why the patient has these concerns, express empathy, but do not feel obligated to answer these types of questions directly at this point in time. Reassure the patient that he is in good hands and that you will answer these questions when more information becomes available. The patient should understand exactly what you know/do not know and can/cannot do at this point in time. This approach creates a sense of trust.

Still others will really be a test of your information-sharing skills. Those may fall under the category of uncertainty because of something the patient does not understand. They will require you to provide the patient with appropriate medical information to minimize uncertainty and then with appropriate reassurances. For example, a patient may say "An ulcer. Oh no. My uncle died from an ulcer." Your response should be to obtain some more details and then explain to the patient how specific management of an ulcer can change the ultimate outcome, while reassuring the patient that this is a good hospital and you will personally manage the care. You are correcting the erroneous belief that everyone with an ulcer dies.

> SPs will always present you with a challenge, but they will not trick you. Everything they do is for a reason, so don't ignore it; just follow their lead.

CHALLENGING SCENARIOS

Patient with severe pain

Acknowledge the patients' pain and explain that you will give medication for it after you have evaluated the cause. Explain that you must first identify the cause in order to give the patient the best medication for the pain. For the pain of an acute abdomen, explain there will be a short delay in providing treatment until you have determined what medication is both needed and safe to be given. Help the patient get into the most comfortable position and save the examination of the painful region for last. Compassionately explain why an exam of this region is of importance; then perform the exam gently and quickly.

Patient who wants treatment without an exam

Mr. Thomas: "I really can't come in to see you. I have no health insurance—can't you just refill my pills? It's only $4 for a month's supply at Wal-Mart. If I do everything you say it will be a hundred times or a thousand times more!"

First, explain to the patient that you understand the current circumstances that have made it difficult to come to see you today. But then stress that there exists the necessity to periodically see patients with chronic medical disorders to review medications and evaluate for complications of the disease.

"I need to see you because you may need different or more medicine. I'll keep your concerns about cost in mind, however I'm going to recommend what is best for your health. I can have you speak with our counselor [social worker], who might be able to help you get health insurance."

Be sure not to promise that the counselor will be able to get the patient health insurance. Have the patient talk to the social worker, if only to see if she can help.

Ms. Gold: "I have a sore throat. My daughter had one a few days ago and her pediatrician gave her antibiotics. I am late for work, so please just give me some antibiotics so I can leave."

Use reassurance and compassion to explain why sometimes an antibiotic can be more harmful than helpful and therefore you want to be sure she needs antibiotics. Explain that doing an examination and performing needed tests is an excellent way to determine if she actually needs them and if so which ones.

Patient who asks if she has cancer

"I know this must be frightening, Mrs. Cheng. I want to understand why you think that you may have cancer. There are many problems other than cancer that can cause you to feel this way. I'll complete my exam, order tests, and have you return in a day or two to present my results with the reason for your symptoms. If it turns out to be something serious I will be there to help you and I have treatments we can try together."

Patient who asks if he is going to die

If asked this question in a case of breaking bad news, such as cancer, respond with honesty and hope–the two "Hs." Be honest about the prognosis and instill realistic hope. Let the patient know of the need to obtain the results of additional tests and to first try some form of treatment and assess the results in order to determine the actual prognosis. Emphasize the outstanding medical and nursing staff with the enormous modern resources available in "this medical center." The doctor is scored on his ability to be honest, reassuring, and empathic. It's a combination of what is said and how it is presented.

Patient who wants more information about a test

Describe tests in lay terms and with honesty, presenting information about discomfort or pain. Emphasize how tests help doctors to solve a patient's problem.

Patient who is angry

A patient may be angry because of a long wait or because other clinicians have been unable to solve his problem. Be prepared to manage these clinical challenges by identifying and discussing them with the patient. Validate the emotions the patient is feeling.

"Ms. White, I can see you are angry. I am sorry that I kept you waiting. I am here now and you have my complete attention." It is usually better not to offer a detailed explanation, such as "The reason that I was late and kept you waiting was that I had to see a patient in the emergency room." These types of explanation often create more rather than less resentment on the part of the patient.

Patient who is verbose

Redirecting the verbose patient to the essence of the history requires patience and finesse. At the right moment, gently interrupt and guide the patient back to a discussion of symptoms. Closed-ended questions are a great way to refocus the discussion.

Patient who is reluctant

How will a patient present with an unclear agenda? One example is the appointment which was made by another person without clarification about the reason for concern, e.g., an adolescent whose mother made the appointment for a "checkup." When faced with this challenge, begin with an open-ended question.

"Why is your mother concerned?"

"Now that you are here, how can I help you?"

"I would really like to help you. If you give me more details about your problem I can help you feel better."

The clinician needs to be patient and kind. If the patient persists in withholding important medical information, consider reassuring about confidentiality.

Patient who asks about HIV or AIDS as a reason for symptoms

Honesty is the key. If you believe it is a remote possibility that the patient is HIV-positive or has AIDS, explain that she is in a low-risk group and this is unlikely to explain the symptoms. If the patient is in a high-risk group with more typical symptoms, be more circumspect, stating the virus may be present but only testing will confirm it. Add that AIDS is now managed as a chronic condition similar to diabetes or hypertension.

Patient with decreased vision or hearing

If a patient has poor vision, tell her where in the room you are sitting and help her with any maneuvers she may need to perform. If the patient has decreased hearing, sit close and speak into the stronger ear.

Patient with intimate partner violence (IPV)

Intimate partner violence is defined as actual or threatened physical, sexual, psychological, and emotional abuse by a current or former partner. IPV is a major challenge because those being abused are ashamed and reluctant to share this information, even with a physician. Patients who experience IPV often present with a somatic symptom that has not been linked to IPV by other physicians. A subtle hint may be if she looks away or becomes teary-eyed when asked about her home or family. Use the SAFE acronym; ask, "Is she concerned about her Safety or the Safety of her children; does she feel Afraid; does she have supportive Friends and/or Family; and, has she made an Emergency plan?" Reassure the patient that you are there to help, by offering medical center resources and support to her and her partner. Remind her that everything is confidential.

Patient who requests that you lie on a form

> Mr. Brown: "Doc, could you just put down on the form that everything is normal? I really need this insurance."

Mr. Brown has just requested that you lie. Apart from not committing insurance fraud, the key to this challenge is to stay calm, non-defensive, and nonjudgmental. Reply with a statement such as, "I'm afraid I can't do that. For now, let us work together to make your health better." If the patient is insistent about what he believes you should include in the form, simply give him back the blank form.

> Mr. Davis: "Please give me the note that states that I am in good health for the job of taxi driver and I'll be on my way. Also Doc, just to let you know, I have the cash on me to pay you."

Apart from not providing the note, the key here is to remain non-defensive and nonjudgmental about the fact that an attempt was just made to bribe you. Just smile, and do what is in the patient's best interest. Be honest and state clearly "I cannot write that note today. I am concerned about your drinking and the falls you have had. I believe you may put yourself and others at risk if you drive a taxi in your current state of health. I would like you to see our alcohol counselor, and we will meet soon after you have the picture of your head. In fact, I'd like to arrange to take the picture now."

PRACTICE CASE

The case that follows gives you the opportunity to test your level of understanding of the 40 skills and shows you examples of how to appropriately incorporate each one of them into any individual case.

Cover the right side of the page and see if you can identify examples of each one of the communication skills from the checklist. If you cannot, review the checklist and explanations and then try again.

PRACTICE CASE: SEVERE ABDOMINAL PAIN

Doorway Information

Opening Scenario

Susan Albright is a 35-year-old woman who comes to the ER complaining of severe abdominal pain.

Vital Signs

T 37.0 C (98.6 F), BP 120/78 mm Hg, HR 100/min (regular), RR 19/min

Pulse oximetry 92% on room air

Examinee Tasks

1. Obtain a focused history.

2. Perform a relevant physical exam. Do not perform rectal, pelvic, genitourinary, female breast, or corneal reflex exam.

3. Discuss your initial diagnostic impression and your workup plan with the patient.

4. After leaving the room, complete your Patient Note.

CIS Skill	Sample Doctor–Patient Interaction
	Sample Doctor–Patient Interaction
1. Knocked	Knock, Knock, Knock
	Patient: Come in
5. Professional appearance	Enter the room wearing a clean white lab coat over professional attire. Notice that the patient is lying on the table in a fetal position facing the right side. When you enter the room her back is to you. She is already draped to the waist. Walk around the table to face the patient.
2. Introduced self 4. Clarified role 3. Patient's preferred title	**Doctor: Hello Ms. Albright? My name is Dr. Levine. I am a doctor at this hospital and will be taking care of you today. I will be asking you questions, examining you, and taking a few notes to be sure I have a record of all the important information. How would you like to be addressed?**
	Patient: Please call me Ms. Albright.
9. Attention and concentration	**Doctor: Ok. Ms. Albright, you look uncomfortable on the examination table. Let me pull out the leg rest so you will be more comfortable while we speak. I will try to be efficient in obtaining all the important information so we can determine what is causing your pain and the best way to treat it.**
11. Eye contact 12. Distance	Sit down on the patient's right side at a 45-degree angle and approximately 2-3 feet away.
15. Elicited chief complaint	**Doctor: What caused you to come see me today?**
	Patient: I am having really terrible stomach pain.
	Doctor: Please point to the pain
	Patient points to right lower quadrant
	Doctor: Thank you. On a scale of 1 to 10, where 10 is the worst pain you have ever had, and 1 is a mild pain, how would you rate this pain?
	Patient: It is terrible. I would call it a 10 out of 10.
38. Empathy and reassurance	**Doctor: I can see you are in a lot of pain. It must have been very difficult for you to even walk into the hospital to come see me today.**
	Patient: Yes, it was. Thank you for noticing and caring.
17. Open-ended question	**Doctor: How would you describe your pain? (What does the pain feel like to you?)**
	Patient: It feels sharp, almost like someone is taking a knife and stabbing me on my side.
16. Timeline of CC	**Doctor: When did it start?**
	Patient: About 6 hours ago
	Doctor: Did it come on suddenly or more gradually?
	Patient: Very suddenly
	Doctor: Is it there all the time, or does it come and go?
	Patient: It is there all the time.
	Doctor: Is it staying the same or getting better or worse?
	Patient: Worse

Doctor: What were you doing when the pain first started? (Can you think of anything that might have brought it on?)

17. Open-ended question

Patient: Nothing in particular. I was just sitting and watching television and all of a sudden it hit me.

Doctor: Does it move anywhere?

Patient: No

Doctor: Did it start where it is now?

Patient: Yes

Doctor: So the pain has always been on your lower right side.

21. Paraphrased

Patient: Yes it has.

Doctor: Ok, so does anything make it worse?

17. Open-ended question

Patient: If I move or take a deep breath, it gets worse.

Doctor: Have you tried anything to make it better?

Patient: I took some Advil I have at home and use once in a while. I thought I would feel fine after that.

Doctor: Did it work at all?

Patient: No

Doctor: Besides the pain, have you been nauseous?

18. Closed-ended question

Patient: Yes. A little.

Doctor: Did you vomit?

18. Closed-ended question

Patient: No

Doctor: So you feel nauseous, but did not vomit. Is that correct?

21. Paraphrased

Patient: Exactly

Doctor: Do you have diarrhea?

Patient: No

Doctor: Have you had a fever?

19. Non-leading question

Patient: I did not take my temperature, but I do not feel warm.

Doctor: How has your appetite been?

Patient: I have not eaten today because the pain is so bad, but I do feel a little bit hungry.

Doctor: Any burning when you urinate?

Patient: No

Doctor: Have you noticed any discharge or liquid coming out of your vagina?

Patient: No

19. Non-leading question

Doctor: Any spotting?

Patient: Yes. When I went to the bathroom before, I noticed a little blood on the tissue.

Doctor: Ok. So when was your last menstrual period?

P: Now that I think about it, I am a little late. It was about 6 weeks ago.

D: Are your periods regular?

P: Yes. Very. I get my period every 28 days.

D: Have you noticed any other symptoms since the pain started?

P: No

27. Transitional phrase

D: Now I am going to ask you some questions about your past health.

P: Okay

D: Have you ever had pain like this before?

P: Never

D: Are you allergic to or have had a strange reaction to any medication?

P: No

D: Are you taking any medication prescribed for you by a physician?

P: No

D: How about anything you may have bought over the counter without a prescription, besides the Advil you mentioned?

P: No

D: Have you ever been hospitalized?

P: Yes, when I was 14 I had surgery for my appendix that burst. And it happened when my parents were away and I was staying at a friend's house.

14. Non-verbal ease

Lean in and nod

38. Empathy and reassurance

D: Sounds like you were pretty sick. Being in a hospital and having surgery in itself would be frightening for a 14 year old. But being alone until your parents could get there must have made it even more difficult for you.

P: Yes it was. Until my parents arrived I felt lonely and scared. And then I was in pain for a while and missed 2 weeks of school.

D: I can understand how upset you must have been

P: Yes I was

D: Have you had any accidents or injuries, especially in the stomach area where you have your pain?

P: No

D: Do you have any medical problems?

P: I once had a urine infection but that is about it. I had some pain then but this feels different.

D: Have you ever had any other surgery besides having your appendix removed?

P: No

D: Recently have you noticed any changes in your urination?

P: No

D: Any blood in your urine?

P: No

19. Non-leading question

D: Any changes in your bowel movements?

P: No

20. Clear and concise questions, one at a time

D: Any changes in the size of your stomach area?

P: No

D: Any changes in your weight?

P: No

D: Have you recently traveled?

P: No

19. Non-leading question

D: Does anyone in your family have the same pain you have?

P: As far as I know, I am the only one who is sick.

D: Any serious illnesses run in your family?

P: Uh. Let me see.

Give patient time to think and do not proceed yet with the next question.

10. Did not interrupt

P: No

D: Have you ever been pregnant?

P: No

D: I am now going to ask you some questions about your sexual history, which is a routine part of the history when a woman has lower abdominal pain. I want you to remember that everything you tell me is confidential. Are you currently sexually active?

27. Transitional phrase
19. Non-leading question

P: Yes I am.

D: How many partners do you have now?

P: Right now just my boyfriend.

D: How many in the past?

P: During the last 10 years, I would say about 20.

D: Do you use condoms?

P: Yes

D: Do you use them consistently?

P: We try to, but we forget many times.

8. Nonjudgmental

D: Thank you.

25. Lay language

D: Do you use any other form of birth control?

P: No

25. Lay language

D: Have you ever had an infection that was transmitted sexually?

P: Yes. Last year I went to my doctor because I had stomach pain,

26. Use of continuer

D: Uh-huh

P: A fever, and a discharge and was told I had PID.

D: Have you ever been tested for HIV, the AIDS virus?

P: I have not.

27. Transitional phrase
19. Non-leading question

D: I am now going to ask you some questions about your habits. Have you ever used tobacco in any form?

P: No

D: Do you drink alcohol?

P: Just socially

10. Repeated question for clarification

D: I want to try and better understand how much alcohol you drink. Can you explain what you mean by drinking alcohol socially?

P: My boyfriend and I have an occasional glass of wine with dinner.

D: Have you ever used recreational drugs?

P: Never. I think drugs are dangerous.

D: Is there anything else about your health that you would like to tell me that I have not asked?

P: No. I think I have told you everything.

27. Transitional phrase

D: Thank you for answering my questions. Now I need to examine you. Before I begin, excuse me while I wash my hands.

6. Care and concern

Wash your hands. (If using hand sanitizer, remember to let the SP see you rubbing your hands together.)

38. Empathy and reassurance

Remember to begin the physical exam in the patient's current position. Do not ask a patient in pain to move more than is necessary.

8. Respect

D: I know you can't see what I am doing so I will explain everything to you.

P: Thank you.

13. Draping
38. Empathy and reassurance

D: While I examine you, your gown will need to be untied, retied, raised, and lowered. Can I help you by doing these things for you?

P: It would be easier if you did it for me. Thank you for offering.

Untie and raise the gown.

D: I need to tap on your back.

Check for CVAT, costovertebral angle tenderness, on the right and left sides.

Lower gown and retie it.

D: I know you are in a lot of pain, but I need to check a few more things that will help me figure out what is wrong. To do this I need you to turn on your back. If it is difficult for you to do this, I can help you turn.

P: Thank you for offering but I can do it myself.

Hold the drape while the patient turns on her back.

D: I am going to take a look at your stomach area.

As agreed upon at the beginning of the physical exam, raise the gown after lowering the drape.

Inspect the abdomen.

D: I need to listen to your stomach.

Auscultate the abdomen in 4 quadrants. Order – RUQ, LUQ, LLQ, RLQ

D: I need to tap on your stomach. Let me know if this causes more pain.

Percuss all 4 quadrants in the same order.

D: I need to press on your stomach. It may hurt but I will be as gentle and quick as possible.

Palpate all 4 quadrants, going last to the RLQ.

P: That really did hurt on my right side.

D: I am so sorry that caused you pain but it gave me some very important information.

I need to press deeper, but I will only press in the areas that did not hurt you. I will not press on your right side again.

P: Thank you.

Palpate deeply the other 3 quadrants.

D: I am going to press on your lower left side. Let me know if it hurts more when I press or when I let go.

P: When you let go.

D: Thank you for allowing me to examine your belly. I know that part of this examination was uncomfortable.

Lower the gown and recover the patient with the drape.

D: Do you want to stay in this position or turn again on your side while I tell you what I am thinking? I want you to be as comfortable as possible while I explain everything to you.

P: I am in a lot of pain and prefer not to move again.

D: First, to summarize, you told me you have had severe pain on your lower right side for 6 hours, that you have had a small amount of vaginal spotting, that your last menstrual period was 6 weeks ago, and that you have had PID in the past. When I pressed on your right lower side it was extremely painful for you. Before I tell you what I am thinking

8. Respect

9. Attention and concentration

6. Care and concern

25. Lay language

7. Connected and purposeful PE

38. Empathy and reassurance

7. Connected and purposeful PE

13. Draping

38. Empathy and reassurance

6. Care and concern

28. Summarized

30. Justified diagnosis

24. What patient thought was going on	**I would like to know what you think is causing your pain. The reason I am asking is that I want to be sure I address all your concerns, explain things properly with enough information, and correct any misinformation you may have.**
	P: A friend of mine had pain like this and her period was also late and she ended up with a pregnancy that ruptured in her abdomen.
29. Diagnostic impression 34. Summarized plan	**D: I do think your problem also is most likely what we call an ectopic pregnancy, which is a pregnancy that is growing outside your womb. To be sure, I am going to order some tests. The first will be a blood test to check if you are pregnant. The second will be a picture of your stomach area to look for the pregnancy. I will get the results as soon as possible and let you know them.**
	P: From my friend I know a pregnancy outside my womb could be very serious and dangerous.
38. Empathy and Reassurance 37. Validated feelings 39. Support system	**D: I understand your concerns. However, there is no need to be unnecessarily concerned at this time. The most important thing is that you are here now at this excellent hospital with very competent doctors. I want to reassure you that I will figure out what is wrong, and if it is serious, we will discuss together and agree on a treatment. I will do everything I can to help you get through this and be there for you until your problem is resolved.**
	Observe patient for reaction.
22. Hidden concern	**D: You still look very worried to me. Is there something else that concerns you that you would be willing to share?**
23. Impact on patient's life	P: Yes. I am afraid I may need surgery, and when I had my appendix removed I was very sick and it took a while to recover. Also, my sister is getting married in 2 weeks and I am her maid of honor.
37. Validated feelings 36. Mutual plan 35. Counseling 32. Asked if patient had questions	**D: Of course that would be concerning to you. If you do end up needing surgery, it will likely be less invasive than your previous surgery. It can be done with a small incision and camera, and you will be home in a day or two and recover much quicker. For now let's take it together one step at a time. Also, I will talk to you in more detail when you are feeling better about using condoms/having safe sex until you are ready to get pregnant. I want to be sure you understand everything that is happening and everything that I have told you. What questions do you have for me?**
	P: None right now.
33. Assessed comprehension	**D: Can I clarify anything I have told you?**
	P: I understand everything so far.
39. Support system	**D: Is there anyone here with you or someone you would like us to call to come be with you?**
36. Mutual plan	P: I was alone when I called the ambulance. So first let's get back my test results and depending what comes next I may call my boyfriend.
31. Assessed need for more Information	**D: Is there anything else that is still concerning you right now?**
	P: No. Now that I understand what may be wrong and what will happen next I am less worried. But, can you give me something for pain?
40. Managed the challenge	**D: I will make sure your test results are returned as quickly as possible. As soon as I know what is causing your pain and I am sure that it is safe, I will give you something for the pain.**
	P: Thank you.
	D: Goodbye.

PART III

Spoken English Proficiency (SEP)

Spoken English Proficiency (SEP) 3

Spoken English Proficiency (SEP) is about understandability in as far as it does not impair or hinder communication. It is not about your accent; it's about how well you and the Standardized Patient (SP) understand each other. The goal is verbally communicating in a way that strengthens the doctor-patient relationship.

COMPONENTS OF SEP GRADING

Five components comprise the grading of SEP:

1. **Pronunciation:** the effect that mispronounced words—not accents—limit comprehension of the questions or comments of the doctor. SPs are specifically trained to listen through accents.

2. **Word choice:** how the words and their component parts combine to form sentences. **Avoid using the same words repeatedly.** Vary your choice of words but keep it simple and use short sentences. The correct use of grammar is also taken into consideration, especially because incorrectly stating something as past when it is present or present when it is past can mislead the patient to be either not concerned or overly concerned.

3. **Doctor's questions and responses being understood by the SP:** the patient does not need to ask the doctor to repeat questions or comments due to lack of understanding.

   If this happens repeatedly, it will affect your SEP score. Do not ignore the SP if he says, "I do not understand." Use different words to ask the same question. For example:

Doctor:	"Do you have angina?"
SP:	"What do you mean?"
Doctor:	"Do you have chest pain?"
SP:	"Oh, yes I do."

4. **SP's questions and responses being understood by the doctor:** the doctor does not need the SP to repeat responses or questions due to lack of understanding.

5. **Listener's effort:** the degree of listening effort that is necessary for the SP to understand the doctor. If you use simpler words, it will be less effort for the SP. Listener's effort can be affected by numerous things:
   - Talked too fast
   - Talked too slow
   - Talked too loud
   - Talked too soft
   - Mumbled

COMPONENTS OF SEP TIME-MANAGEMENT

Doctors are concerned about time management and the 15 minutes that have been allotted for each encounter. SPs are concerned about the time allotment as well.

- SPs have been trained to work within 15 minutes and will adjust their pace so as not to impede you from completing the task required.
- You do not need to speed up your dialogue since that may impair understandability, especially if you have an accent.
- Sometimes responding inappropriately to an SP's question can be interpreted as not understanding or not listening.
  - SPs may use idiomatic phrases or slang whose meaning you do not comprehend. If you are unsure, ask them what they mean.
  - It is not a mark against understandability if you ask for clarity. Do not pretend to understand the SP's meaning. Asking for clarity will strengthen your communication with your SP.
  - There is another skill you can demonstrate if you do not understand your SP. You can paraphrase (repeat back) in your own words what you believe was said. For example:

  > SP: "I've been scratchy and hot for 3 days."
  >
  > Dr. "You've been scratching and had a fever for 3 days?"
  >
  > SP: "No, I've had a sore throat."
  >
  > Dr. "Okay, thank you."

Now you have paraphrased (giving you credit in communication skills) and clarified information to avoid misunderstanding and possible medical error.

RECOMMENDATIONS FOR IMPROVING SEP

If you practice speaking English every day, it will strengthen your confidence, giving you a comfort level which will surely help you to speak more freely with your SP during the encounters.

- Read out loud every day (the newspaper is a good source)
- Record your conversations and then evaluate them. Look to see if you do the following:
  - Mumble
  - Speak too fast or too slow
  - Speak too loud or too soft
  - Do not enunciate words sufficiently

Once you are aware of how you are perceived, record another conversation and notice the improvements.

- Focus and listen without considering your next question or response. This will help to decrease your misunderstandings and strengthen your ability to understand your SP. SEP is about understandability NOT your accent.
- Keep it simple. Use language that is easy to understand and avoid medical jargon.
- Vary your word choices and phrases.

"It is about what you say but, more importantly, it's about **how** you say it."

PART IV

Integrated Clinical Encounter (ICE)

Focused History-Taking 4

This section provides a list of suggested questions to be asked during patient history-taking. Not all of the questions are necessary or relevant to each patient encounter. It is your job, as the physician, to determine the appropriate historical questions to ask. Each question should be focused on the chief complaint, HPI, and aspects of the history related to the CC and HPI. Asking questions that are not relevant to the case will not earn you "more points"; it will only take time away from your ability to ask the appropriate questions.

While you are taking a good focused history from a patient, you need to **listen carefully**. You'll want to listen not only to the words you hear, but also to the tone. You'll also want to observe the patient's **body language**. Be astute in recognizing when the patient looks away, pauses, gets defensive, or becomes angry about a particular question you ask. These behaviors are there for a reason, and you have to be curious enough to dig a little deeper, always in a kind and reassuring manner.

THE MEDICAL INTERVIEW

During the Step 2 CS exam, the primary task is to generate differential diagnoses (hypotheses) with diagnostic and therapeutic plans. The Patient Note should clearly reflect this process, emphasizing primary data from the 15-minute patient encounter.

Introductory (Doorway) Information

Preliminary (introductory) information about the patient is available on the doorway of the examination room with additional copies inside the room and where you write the note. It provides name, age, gender, and the chief concern or complaint. Vital signs are listed:

- Temperature in degrees Fahrenheit and Centigrade (T)
- Blood pressure (BP)
- Heart rate (HR)
- Respiratory rate (RR)

Instructions are given on the tasks needed to complete during the encounter. Unless otherwise stated, it is implied that you will need to perform a physical examination on every SP. A case where a physical examination is not required is a telephone encounter. Read the instructions carefully and begin generating hypotheses that will lead to the correct diagnosis. Generating hypotheses helps save time by narrowing initial questioning to the most likely possibilities. Being a diligent listener will enable the addition or elimination of diagnoses.

PERFORMING THE FOCUSED HISTORY

Chief Complaint (CC)

This is usually a one-sentence description of the patient's reason for the visit.

- In actual practice in the United States, a nurse records this information given from the patient; the nurse writes it on the chart along with the patient's age and sex.
- The nurse then takes the vital signs. (You will accept all vital signs as accurate.)
- The physician reviews this information prior to entering the room. At this point, the physician is already formulating a differential diagnosis, using only the age, sex, chief complaint, and vital signs.
- The physician then enters the room and introduces himself. At this point, a focused history is performed.

An excellent way to start taking the history is to ask an open-ended question. This will give the patient an opportunity to "tell her story." For example:

> "Good morning/afternoon, Mrs. Santos. My name is Dr. Reina. I'm a doctor here in the hospital. I see you are here for chest pain. Can you tell me more about it?"

OR

> "Hello, Mr. Smith, I'm Dr. Wells. I will be taking care of you today. I see that you are here for an ankle injury. Can you tell me more about it?"

Listen closely and focus on what the patient is telling you. The anxiety on the day of the exam may be a strong distraction; however, with practice you will learn to master this skill.

You'll need to **avoid asking questions about something the patient has already stated**. For example, if the patient answers your open-ended question of "Can you tell me more about it?" with "Well, I hurt my ankle yesterday during a 5K race. I twisted it on the curb," and you then ask *when* it occurred, the patient will respond, "Yesterday." Now the patient knows that you have *not been listening*. Remember to listen to his story.

History of Present Illness

After you make your introduction, make the patient comfortable (*offering the drape/dimming the lights/adjusting the table*) and ask your open-ended question, obtain the **history of present illness (HPI)**. If the patient has already told you everything, you may move on to the PMH/Meds/Allergies, etc. This may occur with a simple acute ankle injury.

Most patients, however, do not tell the whole story. They do not know what is important versus what is useless information. It is your job, as the physician, to elicit the important information.

This is the time when a mnemonic may help. Consider a mnemonic to be a road map that will keep you on the path of correct questions. Use it simply as a tool to help you obtain a complete, yet focused, HPI.

Using a mnemonic will help you overcome those stressful moments when you cannot think of any questions to ask. Jot it down on your scrap paper prior to entering the room. If you have memorized it well, simply shooting your eyes down to your notes momentarily to see the mnemonic will help trigger your memory, and help you to ask a question that you may otherwise have forgotten.

SIQOR A6

This mnemonic stands for the following:

Site/Symptom

Intensity/Quantity

Quality

Onset

Radiation

Aggravating Factors

Alleviating Factors

Associated Manifestations

Attributions (what do you think caused this?)

Adaptations (how does it affect your lifestyle?)

Additional Concerns (hidden concerns)

Site

Patients generally refer to bodily location in lay terms and broadly rather than specifically, e.g., "headache," "stomachache," or "backache." The clinician must precisely identify the exact location; it is helpful to have the patient identify the area by pointing.

"Please show me exactly where the pain is."

"Can you point to where it hurts?"

Intensity/Quantity

Questions related to quantity include frequency, size, volume, and number. "How many times did you vomit today?" "How often does the stomach pain occur?" A patient may say that he's been coughing up "a lot of blood," when it turns out to be less than a teaspoon. The intensity of a symptom may be ascertained by asking the patient to use the 1 to 10 scale. The degree of functional impairment is quantified by getting specific details about what a patient can do and for how long.

"If 10 is the worst pain you've ever had, where is this on a scale of 1 to 10?"

Quality

Begin by generally asking what the symptom feels like. If vague terms are used, ask the patient to relate it to a previous similar pain. It is often necessary for the clinician to ask specific questions:

"How would you describe the pain (feeling, discomfort)?"

"Please describe how it feels."

"Tell me what it feels like."

If patient needs prompting:

"Is it a dull ache (sharp, stabbing, burning, pulling, pulsating, cramping, pressure)?"

"Does it come and go?"

"Is the pain there all the time?"

Onset

Dates and times when symptoms first began are consistently the most reliable descriptors of the present illness. Ideally, the patient already gave you the chronology of events after your open-ended question in the beginning. If not, be sure to ask the patient about the very first time the symptom occurred. Patients may minimize early prodromal symptoms that seem unimportant to them but which are very critical diagnostically. Rapidly establish the last time a patient was in a normal state of health; ask one of these questions after inquiring about the chief complaint:

"When were you last in perfect health?"

"When did this first begin?" or "How long have you had this?"

"Have you ever had anything like this before?"

"Can I assume you were in perfect health prior to this?"

Establish the setting in which the patient's illness has developed and the location and time when symptoms occur; this adds precision to the HPI. "Setting" refers to where and when symptoms occur. The frenzy of an office at tax preparation time is obviously relevant when an accountant comes in with burning epigastric pain. For someone who has diarrhea, a recent trip abroad is relevant. Shortness of breath waking a patient in the early hours of the morning is a clue to the presence of congestive heart failure. Exertional chest pain is consistent with coronary artery disease.

"How often do you have this?"

"When do you get these pains (feelings)?"

"When does this occur? What time of day? What are you doing when the pain comes on?"

Radiation

"Questions related to radiation, i.e., movement, are helpful because patients often can tell, in a general way, whether pain or another symptom feels on the surface of their body or deep within."

"Does the pain (or other symptom) move anywhere? Show me where."
(Note: Don't use the word "radiate.")

"Do you feel the pain (or other symptom) anywhere else?"

"Does it ever travel to any other part of your body?"

"Does this pain ever move around?"

Patients are often under stress when they see the doctor, and misunderstandings are frequent. It is helpful to remember common patterns of pain radiation.

Type of Pain	Typically Radiates To
Ischemic chest pain	Arms, neck, back, mandible
Kidney stone	Femoral triangle and testes or vulva
Gallbladder	Posterior right shoulder region
Spleen injury, ruptured ectopic pregnancy	Top of the shoulders (diaphragm irritation)
Testicular torsion	Lower abdomen
Abdominal aortic aneurysm	Back, thoracic region
Pancreatitis	Back, thoracic region
Posterior penetrating gastric ulcer	Back, thoracic region
Lumbar disk herniation	Down lower limb, calf
Pharyngitis pain	Can radiate to ear

Aggravating factors

Questions that elucidate what conditions surround the onset of the symptoms are important. Questions that identify what worsens symptoms provide key information leading you to a more accurate differential diagnosis. Common factors include position, activity level, exertion, relation to food, time of day, and medication use.

"Are you aware of anything that might have brought this on?"

"What happened right before this came on (started)?"

"Did anything unusual happen at that time?"

"Does anything make your pain worse?"

"What makes it worse?"

Alleviating factors

Elucidate the reasons for symptom improvement; this provides additional information. Common factors: position, activity level, exertion, relation to food, time of day, and medication use.

"Does anything make your pain better?"

"What makes it better?"

Associated manifestations

Ask about other specific symptoms associated with the generated hypotheses, i.e., ask a young woman with joint pain about dermatitis and fever if systemic lupus erythematosus is a possible diagnosis.

Asking for "any other symptoms" will have a low yield because SPs are trained to respond with a vague answer: "What do you want to know, doctor?" Your question instead should be:

> "In addition to your headache, have you noticed anything else (e.g., nausea, vomiting, cough, fever, fatigue, loss of appetite, dizziness, cold, sore throat, weakness in your legs, tingling sensation, burning sensation, numbness, sweating)?"

Associated manifestations for cough are fever, sputum, dyspnea, chest pain, and hemoptysis. Associated manifestations for joint pain are redness, swelling, warmth, tenderness, and decreased range of motion

Adaptations

It can be valuable to ask how a patient's symptoms have affected his or her lifestyle. That can be helpful in determining the severity of a symptom. It can also potentially elucidate hidden concerns by the patient or other psychosocial factors. As this type of questioning can demonstrate your concern for the patient's quality of life, it will likely improve the personal rapport you are trying to establish. Your question should be:

> "How does this affect your lifestyle?" or "How does this affect you at work?" or "How does this affect you at home?"

Attribution

Oftentimes patients will have an idea what is causing their symptoms. This can either provide a clue to diagnosis or, if not medically accurate, reveal an area of concern for the patient. Perhaps a patient thinks he has cancer. If that is a diagnostic possibility, then that should be explored. If not, however, you can reassure the patient and alleviate his concern. Your question should be:

> "What do you think is causing your symptoms?"

Additional Concerns

Sometimes patients have additional concerns that have not been uncovered in other lines of questioning. Perhaps they are concerned that they will need to be hospitalized and that they will need to find someone to take care of their children. Other hidden concerns could include wanting pain medication, concerns about having cancer, needing surgery, death, etc. Once you discover a concern, you should address it in an appropriate way. Your question should be:

> "What other concerns do you have?"

Other Components of the Patient's History

During the CS exam, the emphasis is on the HPI. Other aspects of the history are included if they are relevant to the HPI. Details of the present illness will guide one to the related components of the past medical history, family history, social history, and review of systems (symptoms). This flow of questioning allows you to test and refine your diagnostic hypotheses, and provide pertinent positive and negative information to include in the Patient Note.

Past Medical History

Past Medical History (PMH) is a relevant review of systems and symptoms, serious illnesses, hospitalizations, surgeries, medications, diets, weight changes, and sleep patterns.

One mnemonic is **PAMHRFOSS** (ask relevant questions only):

- Previous event similar to the chief complaint
- Allergies (to foods, medicines, plants, animals)
- Medicines (OTC, prescriptions, vitamins, herbs)
- History of hospitalization/illnesses/trauma/surgery (HITS)
- Review of systems
- Family history (focused on problems similar to patient's CC and HPI)
- Ob/Gyn (e.g., last menstrual period [LMP], gravida, para, abortions, infections)
- Sexual history (sexually active, male/female/both, condom use or other method of contraception, STDs, number of partners in past 10 years, sexual function)
- Social history (occupation, home life, exercise, smoking, alcohol, illegal drugs)

Specific Phrases for PAMHRFOSS

PAMHRFOSS: Previous episodes of chief complaint

"Have you ever had this before?"

You may already know the answer to this important question by asking about the symptom's frequency. If a patient has recurrent episodes of an identical headache, the diagnosis is more likely migraine or muscle contraction headache. If it's a new-onset headache in an elder, consider other diagnoses, such as cerebral vascular disease, subdural hematoma, neoplasm, or temporal arteritis.

PAMHRFOSS: Allergies

"Do you have any allergies?"

This is the basic question that must be asked to each patient. All patients need to be asked about allergies to medications. You also need to determine what the symptom is (patients are often confused and believe a side effect is in fact an allergy) to be sure it is an actual allergy. Diarrhea from antibiotics is not an allergy but patients may believe it is.

Patients may also have allergies to foods, plants, animals, or environmental sources. If appropriate for the case, these issues may also need to be addressed. With a 25-year-old woman complaining of a cough for 6 months, for example, you might find out that she moved in with her boyfriend 6 months ago, and that her boyfriend has a cat. Upon further questioning, you find out that she experiences this same type of cough whenever she visits her grandmother (who also has a cat).

If an acute allergic reaction (rash, shortness of breath, anaphylaxis) is in your initial differential diagnosis, a more detailed allergy history is indicated. For example:

"Do you have any allergies to prescription medication?"

"How about any bad reaction to over-the-counter pills or herbal remedies?"

"Any reactions to food?"

"Have you ever had an allergy to shellfish or iodine?"

"Do you have any allergies to animals or plants?"

If you aren't sure you covered all the categories, you may also ask:

"Anything else you can tell me about allergies?"

PAMHRFOSS: Medications

Medications are extremely important. You'll need to ask about medications from each of your patients. There are 3 things to remember:

- Medication (name and why it was prescribed)
- When it was prescribed or stopped (Does that relate to the chief complaint?)
- Is the patient compliant with the medication?
- Is the patient experiencing any common side effects of the medication?

Medication history is inclusive of all of the following categories.

- Prescription medications
- Over-the-counter (OTC)
- Vitamin supplements or herbs
- Oral contraceptives

Some questions which may be important are the following:

"Are you taking any prescription medications?"

"Do you take anything over-the-counter, like Tylenol or aspirin?"

"Do you take oral birth control pills?"

"Do you take any vitamin supplements or herbs?"

"Are you experiencing any side effects from this medication? (If patient is taking a beta blocker, ask about depression and erectile dysfunction; if patient is taking an ACE inhibitor, ask about a dry cough; if patient is taking a calcium-channel blocker, ask about lower extremity swelling.)

For most cases you need only the **drug name**. Dose and frequency may be important if they relate to the chief complaint or your differential diagnosis. For example, a patient complaining of shortness of breath may have been told to take his Lasix (furosemide) 2x a day. He chose to take it only 1x a day because he did not like getting up in the middle of the night to urinate. He is now in congestive heart failure because he was not compliant with his medications. One of the diagnoses you would list is, "*congestive heart failure due to non-compliance of diuretic.*"

If you are not familiar with a drug, ask **why it was prescribed** (this will be a natural lead-in to the past medical history which comes next) or **how it is spelled**.

PAMHRFOSS: History of Hospitalizations, etc.

The PMH will tell you a lot about the patient. A healthy patient who does not take any medications and sees his physician regularly is most likely a healthy patient. There is no need to ask about specific diseases.

The HITS can be divided into 4 components:

- Hospitalizations (**H**)
- Major illness (**I**)
- Significant trauma (**T**)
- Surgical history (**S**)

Hospitalizations

If a hospitalization was recent, new symptoms or complaints may be a complication or progression of the problem.

"Have you ever been hospitalized?"

"What was the problem that caused the hospitalization, and approximately how long were you hospitalized?" (if relevant, What was the treatment?)

Major Illness

Ask about specific diseases when appropriate. Many heart disease patients forget they also have diabetes.

Many patients have been told in the past that their blood pressure was too high, but they never followed up with a physician.

Trauma

"Have you ever had any major injuries?"

Surgery

"Have you ever had any surgeries?" (Because many surgeries are done on an outpatient basis, you cannot assume the patient has not had surgery if she denies hospitalization. If told of any surgeries when asking about hospitalizations, be sure to say, "aside from what you told me already?" or the SP will think you're not listening.)

PAMH<u>R</u>FOSS: Review of Systems (ROS)

Review of systems is the time to ask screening questions. It is the time to see if there are other major problems that you have not yet uncovered. You can ask about any organ system that you feel is relevant, but focusing on 3 systems is sufficient for most cases. Depending on the relevance, select 3 of the following:

HEENT

"Do you get headaches?"

"Have you had any visual changes?"

"Do you have any trouble with your ears?"

"Do you get nosebleeds?"

"Do you have any throat pain or soreness?"

"Do you have any difficulty swallowing?"

Constitutional (an especially important category to ask because it helps you understand if the problem is systemic, i.e., an infection or cancer)

"Have you been having fevers?"

"Have you been feeling warmer or colder than usual?"

"Do you sweat or have chills at night?"

"Has there been any change in how much you sleep or eat?"

"Are you feeling fatigued or weak?"

Increased sleep may be due to depression, hypothyroidism, sleep apnea, medication, or illegal drugs.

Decreased sleep may be due to anxiety, depression, hyperthyroidism, medication, illegal drugs, or mania.

Respiratory

"Do you get shortness of breath?"

"Do you wheeze?"

"Do you cough up sputum?"

Cardiac

"Do you ever feel your heart beating rapidly (have palpitations)?"

"Do you have any trouble with your heart?"

"Do you have any difficulty exercising, walking up stairs, doing your regular activities?"

Gastrointestinal

"Have you had any change in your bowel habits?"

"Do you have any trouble with diarrhea or constipation?"

"Has your weight changed any?"

"Have your eating habits changed in any way?"

Note: It is common for vegans to develop vitamin B12 deficiency.

Have prepared by Test Day the short differential for weight gain and weight loss:

Weight gain: depression, hypothyroidism, an edematous state (heart failure, chronic liver disease, or chronic renal failure), and eating disorder (not common as a CS exam case)

Weight loss: neoplasm, depression, anxiety, hyperthyroidism, chronic illness, use of an illegal drug, and eating disorder

Urinary

"Have you had any changes in your urinary habits?"

"How often do you urinate?"

"How many times do you get up at night to urinate?"

"Do you have any burning with urination?" "Any blood?"

"Is the stream weak?"

"Do you ever lose control of your bladder?"

If the chief complaint is dysuria, all of the questions are asked in the HPI.

Musculoskeletal

"Do you have joint pain anywhere in your body?"

PAMHRFOSS: Family History

The family history is relevant only if the diagnosis you are considering has a genetic or familial component. Do not ask the family history if it isn't relevant. If you do need a family history, make a transitional statement first. "Now I will ask you about your family's health." Then, ask as many of the following questions as appropriate.

"Does anyone in your family have what you have?"

"Does anyone in your family have high blood sugar? High blood pressure?"

"Does anyone in the family have any serious illness?"

If a serious illness or death is mentioned in the family history, a simple compassionate statement is always appreciated by the patient: "I am sorry to hear that."

PAMHRFOSS: Obstetrical and Gynecology History

Relevance to the HPI is the key for asking questions about the obstetrical and/or gynecological history. Remain sensitive about a patient's culture and privacy. Iron-deficiency—the most common reason for anemia—is related to the combined effects of menses and pregnancy.

Obstetrical History

How to determine a patient's GPA status:

G = number of times pregnant

Ask, "How many times have you been pregnant?"

P = number of live births; any pregnancy that ended at 20 weeks or later, even if it did not result in a live birth

Ask, "How many times have you given birth?"

A = any pregnancy that ended prior to 20 weeks, including miscarriages, induced abortions, and ectopic pregnancies

Ask, "Have you had any miscarriages or elective abortions?"

Gynecological History

Components of a comprehensive gynecological history are the following:

- Regularity of menses
- Cramps/pain with menses
- Flow amount (can be assessed by determining number of sanitary pads/tampons used per day) and number of days the flow is heavy)
- Cycle length
- Age of menarche/age of menopause
- Spotting between cycles
- Vaginal discharge
- Last Pap smear

Suggested questions are:

"When was your last menstrual period?"

"Was it normal?"

"Any change in your period recently?"

"Do you have a period every month?" "How long between periods?"

"Are you regular? How many days do you use pads or tampons? How many pads or tampons per day?" (Note: In the United States, average total number for a menstrual flow is 12/menses.)

"When did you start having periods? When did you stop menstruating? Have you had any bleeding or spotting since menopause?"

"Any mood swings or irritability around your period? Anything else?"

PAMHRFOSS: Sexual History

The sexual history or parts of the sexual history are needed only if relevant to the case, especially if you think the patient could have a sexually transmitted disease, could be pregnant, or, if female, has lower abdominal pain. Also, ask yourself if sexual function could be compromised by the diagnoses you are considering. Examples of this are angina precipitated by sexual intercourse or erectile dysfunction caused by depression, diabetes, or beta blockers.

It is important that you not be nervous when asking these questions. Practice them over and over until you can ask them without embarrassment.

Standard sexual history questions are the following:

"Are you sexually active?"

"Are your partners men, women, or both?"

"How many sexual partners have you had in the last 6 months? in the last 10 years?"

"Do you use birth control, and if so, what type? always or sometimes?

(if a female patient takes oral contraceptives, you should still need ask about use of condoms because OCPs do not protect against sexually transmitted diseases)

"Have you ever had a sexually transmitted infection?"

"Have you ever been tested for HIV or AIDS?"

"Do you have any concerns about sexual function?"

Be sure to listen to the patient's answer and consider that most of these questions may not be needed, unless they somehow relate to the chief complaint or your differential diagnosis.

PAMHRFOSS: Social History

The social history is a unique part of the history. It is important because some social behaviors increase the patient's risk for certain diseases. Smoking for many years increases a patient's risk for chronic obstructive lung disease, lung cancer, coronary artery disease, peripheral vascular disease, abdominal aortic aneurysm, and cerebral vascular disease. Long-term alcohol abuse increases a patient's risk for liver disease.

This is also the time to ask about sick contacts (for instance, if the patient has a sore throat, find out if anyone she lives with also has a sore throat).

The social history also helps strengthen the physician/patient bond. The patient will feel that you are really taking an interest in him. You will rarely need to take a complete social history.

However, the following components may be important, depending on the chief complaint and your postulated differential diagnosis.

- Tobacco
- Alcohol
- Recreational drugs
- Diet
- Exercise
- Occupation/work life
- Home life

Ask, when appropriate, a question about intimate partner violence: "I ask my patients whether there are problems or conflicts at home?"

Depending on the case, ask about parts or all of the social history.

Tobacco

An efficient way to determine smoking history is to ask the following:

Doctor: "Have you ever used tobacco products?"

Patient: "Yes, I smoked for 30 years and stopped last week. I also stopped using cigars and chewing tobacco last week."

Incorrect: "Do you smoke?"

If you asked the same patient, "Do you smoke?" he may reply "No," because he quit last week. In that case, you would miss the entire tobacco history!

If the patient has a disease that is caused or exacerbated by smoking, it is helpful to know the total lifetime exposure.

Pack-Years = (number of packs per day) x (number of years)

So 20 pack-years could mean 20 years at 1 pack per day or 40 years at 1/2 pack per day.

If the chief complaint is that the patient wants to receive smoking cessation help, you will need to know when he started to smoke, what he has tried to do in the past to stop, and what methods of quitting have and have not been successful for him.

Alcohol

Ask about alcohol use if it is appropriate for the case. An effective way to ask about alcohol use is the following:

Doctor: "Do you drink alcohol?"

Patient: "Yes."

Doctor: "What do you like to drink and how much do you drink in a typical day?"

Quantify the number of alcoholic beverages your patient drinks in a day—it doesn't matter if it is beer, whisky, vodka, or wine. If a man or woman drinks one glass of wine (or anything else) daily with dinner, you do not need to ask any further questions. These patients do not need counseling and they certainly do not need to be asked the CAGE questions.

If, however, you suspect alcohol abuse (a man who consumes more than 2 drinks a day OR a woman who consumes more than 1 drink a day OR anyone who binges on the weekends), then the CAGE questions would be appropriate to determine if the patient is abusing alcohol.

CAGE Questionnaire

Ask the following questions if you suspect the patient has a problem with alcohol:

1. "Have you ever felt you should Cut down on your drinking?"

2. "Have people Annoyed you by criticizing your drinking?"

3. "Have you ever felt bad or Guilty about your drinking?"

4. "Have you had a drink first thing in the morning to steady your nerves or get rid of a hangover? (Eye opener)?"

Two positive responses suggest the patient may have an alcohol abuse problem. Counseling and support services should be offered to the patient.

Courtesy of Dr. John Ewing. "Detecting Alcoholism: The CAGE Questionnaire, JAMA 252: 1905-1907, 1984."

Recreational (Illegal) Drug Use

The correct way to ask about drug use is the following:

Doctor: "Do you or have you ever used recreational drugs?"

Patient: "Yes."

Doctor: "What do you use?"

Patient: "Cocaine, when I can get it."

Doctor: "How do you take it?"

Patient: "I smoke it."

Doctor: "When did you last use?"

Patient: "About 20 minutes ago."

If a patient uses recreational drugs, you should identify the specific substances, routes used (ingested, smoked, snorted, or IV), and date of last use. A patient may be willing to quit; ask if an attempt has been made and what method has been tried.

SPs do make an effort to avoid using slang words in their speech. If you don't understand the street name of a recreational drug, it is fine to ask the patient.

Patient: "I use coke sometimes."

Doctor: "Is that cocaine?"

Patient: "That's right, Doc."

Common Names for Recreational Drugs

Alcohol: booze, brews, brewskis

Amphetamines: speed, crank, crystal meth

Cannabis: hash, hashish, dope, pot, reefer, bud, ganja, weed, grass

Cocaine: blow, coke, toot, nose candy, crack

Downers: generic street name for benzodiazepines or barbiturates

Heroin: horse, brown sugar, smack

Phencyclidine: PCP, angel dust

Anabolic steroids: 'roids

Exercise

Asking about exercise is appropriate when a patient comes in for a general checkup or a periodic physical exam, but not when the visit is for an acute problem.

Occupation/Work Life

A patient's occupation and occupational exposures may be clues to the cause of symptoms. A high stress level at work can be the foundation for symptoms. A coal miner who is short of breath may have pneumoconiosis.

Marital Status/Home Life

Asking about home life provides noteworthy social information, particularly if you suspect intimate partner violence:

> Doctor: "Do you live alone or with others?" (If "with others" but the patient doesn't clarify, ask what their relationship is.)
>
> Patient: "My wife and our 3 teenagers."
>
> Doctor: "Is there any stress at home?"
>
> Patient: "No, just the usual stuff with kids."

THE PEDIATRIC HISTORY

Infants and children do not participate in the CS exam. A parent, grandparent, or guardian will present the child's history in person or through a telephone conversation. Review all components of the chief complaint, HPI, and relevant PMH with the parent or guardian, as noted in previous sections.

In addition to the standard PMH, review the specialized pediatric history below.

Prenatal

- "How was the mother's health during her pregnancy with the child?"
- "Were there any infections, illnesses or excessive vaginal bleeding?"
- "Did the mother smoke, drink, take medications or use recreational drugs?"
- "Did the mother go for routine prenatal checkups?"

Birth

- "Was the baby born prematurely or was the baby full-term?"
- "How much did the baby weigh?"
- "What type of delivery did the mother have? Was it a normal spontaneous vaginal delivery (NSVD) or an operative delivery (forceps, vacuum extraction, or cesarean section)?"
- "What were the baby's Apgar scores, if known?"

Neonatal

- "Did the child have any medical problems at birth?"
- "Was the child blue (cyanotic)? Did the child have breathing problems (respiratory distress)? Was the child's skin yellow (jaundice)? Was the child shaking (seizures)? Did the child have an infection?"

Note

Since a physical exam will never be performed for a pediatric case, the first thing in the diagnostic workup section of the patient note will always be the physical exam required to complete the medical evaluation.

- "Did the child go to the well-baby nursery or intensive care nursery?"
- "How long did the mother and baby stay in the hospital after delivery?"

If the parent is not sure of the exact medical problems but knows some existed, then ask about length of stay. Typical length of stay after a vaginal delivery is 2 days and slightly longer after a cesarean section. A prolonged hospitalization confirms either complications or extreme prematurity (as long as it was not for maternal indications).

Feeding

- "Was the child breastfed or bottle-fed?"
- "Were there any feeding problems?"
- "If breastfed, at what age was it stopped?"
- "If bottle-fed, what formula was used?"
- "When did the child start eating solid food?" (Should occur at 6 months.)
- "How is the child's current appetite?"
- "Is the child taking pediatric multiple vitamins?"
- "Does the child have any food allergies?"

Development

- "Has the child gained weight appropriate to growth charts?"
- "Has there been any sudden loss or gain of physical growth?"
- Look for changes in the pattern of growth and deviations from the child's own trajectory of growth.
- Look for deviations from what is typical for other members of the child's family.
- "Has the child achieved developmental milestones?"

The 5 domains of child development are gross motor, fine motor, speech and language, cognitive and social/emotional development. As the time limitations of the CS exam do not allow for a review of all milestones, inquire about a few representative ones.

- "Did your child recognize you by 2 months?"
- "Did your child laugh by 4 months?"
- "Did your child roll over by 7 months?"
- "Did your child say "mama" or "dada" by 9 months or other 1-2 words by 12 months?"
- "Did your child walk alone by 18 months?"
- "Was your child toilet trained by age 3?"
- "Did your child dress herself and know her colors by age 4?"
- "Did your child print his first name and follow rules by age 5?"
- "If the child is school aged, has the child made the appropriate progress in school, including interaction with peers?"

Routine Care

- "Does the child go for routine checkups?"
- "When was the last checkup?"
- "Are the child's vaccinations or shots up-to-date?"
- "Were there any unexpected reactions?"

THE PATIENT WITH A PSYCHIATRIC DIAGNOSIS

Psychiatric History

Fatigue consistently ranks among the most common presenting complaints to physicians in all practice settings.

Many studies have revealed that 40–80% of patients complaining of persistent fatigue in a clinical setting meet the criteria for a psychiatric disorder. In light of these findings, it is recommended that physicians consider underlying psychosocial problems as part of their differential diagnoses. This is equally important on the Step 2 CS exam.

A high-yield CS diagnosis to consider with a chief complaint of fatigue is **major depressive disorder**.

The patient may state any of the following:

- "I feel overwhelmingly tired all the time."
- "Everything I need to do is an effort."
- "I am not my usual self."
- "I feel totally exhausted, worn out, drained, or run-down."
- "I don't have the energy to get through my typical days."

Begin by using the standard history mnemonic.

- **Q-Quality**: What do you mean by fatigue? Tell me more details about your chief complaint.
- **Intensity**: Ask about the impact on activities of daily living, such as the ability to care for oneself (cook, clean, dress, hygiene) and function appropriately at work and in social situations.
- **O-Onset**: When did it start? (duration of 2 weeks for MDD) Did it come on suddenly or more gradually? Is it constant or intermittent? If intermittent, what is the typical frequency and duration? Is the course staying the same or getting better or worse? Was there a precipitating factor connected to the onset, such as trauma, divorce, bereavement, financial problems, loneliness, or a move? Why are you seeking treatment at this particular time?
- **A, A-Aggravating and Alleviating factors**: What makes it worse? What makes it better? Fatigue that is aggravated by exertion and alleviated by rest is more frequently associated with physical diseases.

If you suspect that the patient has MDD, ask the following questions:

- S: increased or decreased sleep, early morning awakening
- I: decreased interest in activities (anhedonia)
- G: feeling of guilt, worthlessness, hopelessness, regret
- E: decreased energy or fatigue (The CC for this case)
- C: decreased concentration, difficulty making decisions
- A: appetite increase with weight gain or decrease with weight loss
- P: decreased or increased psychomotor activity
- S: suicidal ideation

Note

Expect to find fatigue as the stated chief complaint for multiple cases.

Note

Be prepared for a psychiatry case if you see one of the following doorway tasks:

- "Do not perform a physical exam"

- "Perform a relevant physical exam" but then the SP is wearing street clothes rather than a hospital gown

For a diagnosis of MDD, the patient must have at least 5 of the symptoms, and must include either depressed mood or anhedonia. Other somatic symptoms may be headache, abdominal pain, or musculoskeletal pain.

Remember to ask all the associated symptoms connected to the other likely differential diagnoses being considered for the patient note. For example, hypothyroidism is a good choice as a differential for MDD. Ask about weight gain, cold intolerance, dry cool skin, brittle hair, constipation, slow speech, muscle weakness, and hoarseness.

Focused previous medical history:

- P: Have you ever felt like this before? (MDD tends to be recurrent)
- Are you allergic to any medications?
- M: Are you taking any prescription or over-the-counter medications? (beta-blockers, alpha interferon, isotretinoin, and corticosteroids have depression as a side effect)
- H: Have you ever been hospitalized (specifically) for a previous psychiatric indication?
- Do you have any known history of diseases and especially psychiatric illnesses? If so, were you given any psychological or pharmacological treatments?
- T: Trauma such as child abuse which may be a risk factor?
- S: Surgery?
- F: Does anyone in your family have a similar symptom of fatigue? Is there a family history of any psychiatric disorders? (it can be familial)
- O: Obstetrics (recent pregnancy suggests post-partum depression)
  - Onset should be during pregnancy or within 1 month of the birth and continue beyond 2 weeks
  - Mother may have negative or ambivalent feelings toward the infant
  - Self-limited baby blues typically has an immediate onset and does not last more than 2 weeks
- S: Sexual (decreased libido may be associated with depression)
- S: Social: Do you use tobacco products, drink alcohol, or use recreational drugs? (excessive alcohol intake, as well as use of drugs, can cause fatigue and affect mood)
- Diet and Exercise (poor dietary choices and excessive exercise can cause fatigue)
- Home and Work:
  - Where do you live? With whom do you live? Are you currently employed?
  - Do you feel stressed at home or at work?
  - Remember that victims of domestic violence may present with fatigue and depressed mood.
- Have you withdrawn from relationships and no longer participate in work, family, and leisure activities?
- Recent loss of a job or relationship and change in family and friend social network with isolation could be a relevant trigger for the case.
- What were your personality and social interactions prior to the onset of your current symptoms?

At first glance, when taking a history in CS psychiatry cases, the reported information may seem pertinent to multiple high yield diagnoses. A significant number of history findings can typically be used as justifications in patient notes for many of them. Fatigue, changes in sleep and eating, irritability, anxiety, inability to focus and concentrate, diminished capacity to function in work and social situations, to name of few, can be relevant for many psychiatry differential diagnoses.

The following review of common CS psychiatry disorders will help the examinee identify differentiating facts and therefore enable the selection of the most likely primary diagnosis for each scenario.

Bipolar Disorder

With bipolar disorder, patients experience **at least 1 manic episode lasting at least 1 week** and possible depressive episodes. Manic episodes are characterized as periods of high energy; euphoria; decreased need for sleep; increased goal directed activity; risky behaviors such as excessive spending; gambling and hyper-sexuality; irritability; distractibility and easy frustration. Patients may report that friends recently observed their being more talkative than usual and/or very hyper.

Adjustment Disorder

Patients with this disorder report an **identifiable psychosocial stressor** connected to the onset of symptoms such as overwhelming anxiety, irritability, and depression. This results in a decrease in work and social performance. The patient's response is in excess of what would typically occur in response to a particular stressor, such as a friend moving away or a relationship ending. Look for onset within 3 months of stressor and duration of up to 6 months once the stressor is resolved.

Generalized Anxiety Disorder

With generalized anxiety disorder, patients experience **excessive, uncontrollable and unrealistic worries** about **normal life situations**. They may describe themselves as being out of control, and feeling on edge or unable to relax. Symptoms include fatigue, muscle tensions, sleep disturbances, poor concentration, irritability, restlessness, hyperarousal, and hypervigilance. Other symptoms of anxiety may include diaphoresis, dyspnea, palpitations and dizziness. There may be a deterioration in both occupational and social functioning. Look for a **duration of 6 months** and the absence of a connection to a specific focus or event which will be present in specific anxiety disorders such as social anxiety disorder.

Panic Attack

With panic attack, patients experience **sudden unexpected anxiety episodes** lasting for several **minutes**. Autonomic symptoms include hyperventilation, dyspnea, chest pain, palpitations, diaphoresis, tremors, nausea, dizziness, paresthesias and heat or cold sensation. For a duration of at least 1 month, the patient may experience concern and fear about future attacks that may lead to a gradual limitation of activities. They may communicate a fear of going crazy or having a life threatening disease. The presence of agoraphobia may be noted, as the patient will avoid public places where it may be difficult to escape in the event of panic symptoms.

Social Anxiety Disorder

Social anxiety disorder is an **excessive and irrational fear of social situations**, which leads people to avoid them. The patient fears being humiliated or embarrassed by those present. The standardized patient may report avoiding public speaking or even eating in public. This pattern of behavior interferes with the patient's ability to function in both professional and personal environments. Symptoms of anxiety may be reported.

Post-Traumatic Stress Disorder

Post-traumatic stress disorder (PTSD) develops in response to the patient experiencing or witnessing a traumatic event, such as death or a serious injury. The SP may report flashbacks or nightmares, during which time the event is re-experienced. In response, the patient will avoid any reminders of the event and may actually be unable to recall many of the specific details. Symptoms include anger, anxiety, hypervigilance, impulsiveness, difficulty focusing and concentrating, sleep disturbances, and inability to function in both professional and social situations. Look for duration of symptoms >**1 month**.

Acute stress disorder is the correct diagnosis if duration of symptoms <**1 month** and **onset is within 1 month of stressor**.

Schizophrenia

Schizophrenia is a thought disorder that results in impaired judgment and inappropriate behavioral responses to real world situations. The patient may report a history of arrests secondary to aggressive actions such as assault, in the context of **paranoia, hallucinations**, or **delusions**. The patient may also communicate information such as being watched by neighbors, the police, or even the government, and verifies the validity of these statements by saying "the voice in my head told me it was true." Look for continued impaired functioning in either work or social environment, as well as in self-care, for duration of symptoms **6 months**, with at least **1 month of active symptoms**. Multiple abnormalities will be detected on the psychiatric mental status physical exam.

- Schizophreniform disorder is the correct diagnosis if duration >**1 month but <6 months**.
- Brief psychotic disorder is the correct diagnosis if duration <**1 month** and the patient then returns to baseline.

Paranoid personality disorder should be considered in the absence of delusions and hallucinations.

Focused Physical Exam 5

The physical exam is sharply focused on the patient's chief complaint, the symptoms identified during the HPI, and your generated hypotheses. To perform a targeted physical exam, you must have a well-considered differential diagnosis and knowledge of which physical findings would be expected for each condition included in the differential. Because of the time constraint imposed by the Step 2 CS, it is critical that you keep your exam focused.

GENERAL POINTS

- Standardized patients (SPs) are diligently trained to simulate the illness being portrayed.
  - Physical findings can be imitated and enhanced by the application of stage makeup.
  - Actors with actual abnormalities, as well, can be placed into the setting of the case. A person with a known cardiac murmur can reliably simulate a patient with infective endocarditis.
    - Therefore, consider all detected abnormalities as real.
- You are **not permitted** to do the following exams: female breast, pelvic, rectal, genital (including evaluation for inguinal hernia), corneal reflex, or throat swab.
  - Instead, list a necessary exam for any of these regions in your diagnostic plan.
  - If synthetic models are used for these exams, instructions will be provided.
- At the appropriate time, tell the patient you are going to conduct the exam, wash your hands or use hand sanitizer, and proceed.
  - Drape the patient with care; never examine through clothing.
  - Make sure the patient removes socks if you are going to examine the feet.
  - Before you examine a region, let the patient know what you will do, e.g., "I am now going to examine your ears."
- For women, ask the patient to assist you when examining the anterior thorax, heart, and lungs.
  - She can lift her breast to enable you to look for and palpate the apical impulse. Instruct the patient to move her bra or lift her breast.
- If the patient is fearful of an exam due to pain, say, "I know you are in pain, but it's important that I examine you. I'll be gentle and quick and I'll let you know exactly what I'm going to do before I do it."
  - Assist the patient into the best position to help relieve some of the pain (i.e., adjust the table up or down).
- It's perfectly appropriate to ask questions about the history during the physical exam.
- Allow 3 to 4 minutes to perform the physical exam. Your main objective is to thoroughly examine the target area and use the remaining time to examine other areas related to your differential.

EXAMPLE PHYSICAL EXAM

A 73-year-old man presents with left-sided chest pain, nausea, diaphoresis, and palpitations.

Differential diagnosis:

- Acute coronary syndrome
- Pulmonary embolus
- Pneumothorax
- Pneumonia
- Costochondritis

Physical exam checklist:

- ❏ Washed hands prior to exam
- ❏ Palpated left chest wall for reproducible tenderness
- ❏ Looked and palpated for apical impulse
- ❏ Auscultated heart in all 4 cardiac areas (while sitting upright and while laying down at 30-45°)
- ❏ Examined lungs (6 areas in back, 4 areas in front)
    - A. Tactile vocal fremitus
    - B. Percussion
    - C. Auscultation
- ❏ Inspected for JVD
- ❏ Evaluated peripheral pulses
- ❏ Inspected calves for swelling, tenderness
- ❏ Palpated lymph nodes

In this case, the cardiac and lung exams were relatively thorough because cardiac and pulmonary diseases were high on the differential diagnosis list. A neurologic exam was not necessary (especially if, during the history-taking section, the patient denied having any numbness/tingling or weakness).

- In your Patient Note, comment on the general appearance. If the patient was visibly uncomfortable due to the left-sided chest pain, you could write, "Patient uncomfortable secondary to pain."
- Accept the vitals as being correct. Do not repeat them unless you are instructed to do so by the Doorway Information.
- Try to start with the most relevant organ system first, and do it completely. Then, examine other organ systems that are relevant to the differential diagnosis.

FOCUSED EXAMS BY SYSTEM

HEENT and Neck/Thyroid Exams

Do HEENT and Neck exams when there are complaints of:

- Headache
- Head trauma
- Ocular problems (visual disturbance, eye pain)
- Ear problems (tinnitus, vertigo, hearing loss)
- Nasal problems (rhinorrhea, epistaxis, sinus pain)
- Pharyngitis, voice changes, jaw pain
- Fatigue

Perform only the relevant components of the HEENT and Neck/Thyroid exams depending on your differential diagnosis. To conduct the exam, do the following:

Head

- Inspect for trauma, scars, hair changes, other relevant abnormalities
- Palpate for tenderness

Eyes

- Inspect sclera/conjunctiva for color; pupils for size, shape, and symmetry
- Inspect visual acuity with the Snellen chart
  - Ask patient to cover left eye and read the smallest possible line on the chart; repeat for right eye, asking patient to read the smallest line possible backward
- Peripheral vision (visual fields):
  - Ask patient to cover the eye that is not being tested; it is crucial that patient look straight ahead and not at your fingers
  - Rapid method: bisect the pupil horizontally and vertically, creating 4 small quadrants
    - First, wiggle your fingers in both upper (superior) quadrants, then in both lower (inferior) quadrants, asking patient to point to which fingers are moving
    - Now repeat the same maneuver with other eye, checking all 4 visual fields
- Check extraocular movements
  - Ask patient to look straight ahead and follow your index finger; make a wide "H" in the air, and ask patient to follow with the eyes
  - This will check all of the extraocular movements and check for nystagmus
- Pupillary light reflex: check direct response (constriction of the illuminated pupil), as well as consensual response (constriction of the opposite pupil)
- Check accommodation: it is easier to view the pupil dilate rather than constrict because most irises are dark brown
  - Place your finger 12 inches from eye, then ask patient to look into the distance; the pupil will dilate

- Inspect the fundus:
  - Dim lights in room
  - Remove ophthalmoscope from holder and make sure unit is turned on
  - Shine light on your hand, adjusting light color and diameter (set lenses at zero)
  - Ask patient to stare at a point on the wall
    - Coming in from the side and holding instrument in right hand, use your right eye to examine patient's right eye
    - Then hold instrument in left hand and use your left eye to examine patient's left eye

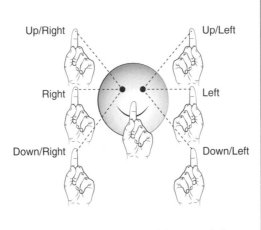

Extraocular Movements and Accommodation

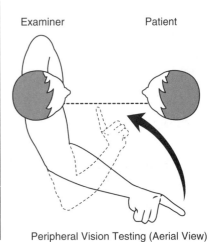

Peripheral Vision Testing (Aerial View)

Ears

- Inspect the external ear for abnormalities. Palpate the ear, tragus, pinna, and mastoid area for tenderness.
- Inspect the canal and drums.
  - Remove the otoscope from its holder and turn light on.
  - Put on a new speculum; secure it tightly
  - Gently move pinna superiorly (up) and posteriorly (back); this maneuver straightens the cartilaginous section of the canal
  - Gently, by direct visualization, place tip of speculum into the external auditory meatus
  - Gently introduce the speculum while looking through the lens; once the tip is in the ear canal, do not move the otoscope in any plane as that would cause discomfort to the patient
- Do Rinne and Weber tests only if there is hearing loss on history or physical exam.
  - **Rinne**: Place vibrating tuning fork on mastoid process. When patient no longer hears it, move to external ear and determine if patient can still hear the vibration.
  - **Weber**: Place vibrating tuning fork on center of forehead. Check if sound is equal in both ears.

Use of a Tuning Fork to Determine the Cause of Hearing Loss:
Sensorineural Versus Conductive

Diagnosis	Hearing	Rinne	Weber
Normal	Normal	AC > BC	Equal
Conductive loss	Decreased	BC > AC	Louder on the side with the hearing loss
Sensorineural loss	Decreased	AC > BC	Louder on the normal side; softer on the side with the hearing loss

Nose

- Inspect the external nose
- Palpate nose and sinuses (frontal, ethmoid, and maxillary)
- Inspect nasal turbinates with a light source

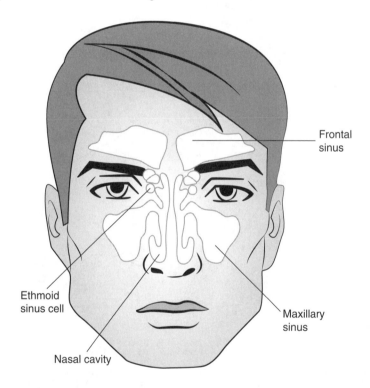

Frontal sinus

Ethmoid sinus cell

Maxillary sinus

Nasal cavity

Oral Cavity and Throat

- Inspect with a light source
- Inspect the tonsillar fossae and oropharynx; gently use a tongue depressor, keeping it anteriorly to prevent a gag reflex
- Examine oral cavity, tongue, and oropharynx

Neck Exam

- Ask the patient to untie the gown, moving it inferiorly to below the clavicles. Explain to the patient the necessity for improving exposure.
- Inspect the neck for any visible abnormalities.
- If there are musculoskeletal symptoms, examine the muscles of the neck for tenderness and perform a range of motion.

- Examine the neck for lymphadenopathy:
  - Using both hands simultaneously, palpate with the finger pads of the 3 middle fingers while moving in a circular motion. Begin in the posterior neck inferior to the occiput (occipital nodes), moving to the mastoid processes (postauricular nodes), anterior to pinnae (preauricular nodes), inferior to mandible (submandibular nodes), and inferior to chin (submental nodes).
  - Move fingers along the sternocleidomastoid muscle (superficial cervical nodes), along the anterior edge of the trapezius (posterior cervical nodes), and in the angle formed by the sternocleidomastoid and clavicle (supraclavicular nodes).

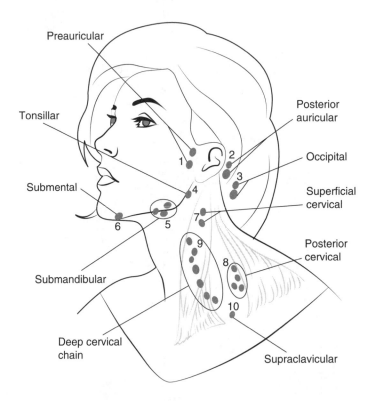

Thyroid Exam

- Ask patient to swallow (offer water if needed); observe thyroid gland movement.
- Go around the back (or stay in front, whichever you prefer), and using the finger pads of your 3 middle fingers, palpate the thyroid gland below the cricoid cartilage on both sides
- Ask patient to swallow again, feeling the thyroid gland slip under your fingers.
- Hold the left side of the thyroid gland stationary while you palpate the right. Check for nodules, tenderness, or enlargement. Then do the same on the other side.
- Check for associated abnormalities like skin, hair, reflexes, and heart rhythm changes. Also examine for myxedema and tremor.

Suggested Phrasing for HEENT Exam

Action	Suggested Phrasing	Comments
Palpation of head	"I need to press lightly on your head."	
Palpation of sinuses	"Now let me press lightly on your face."	
Palpation of ears	"Now I'll press around your ears."	
Palpation of lymph nodes	"I will press on your neck."	"Lymph nodes" is medical terminology.
Ophthalmoscope Eyes	"Please pick a point on the wall. I am going to check your eyes."	
Otoscope Ears Nose Oral cavity and throat	"I am going to look inside your ears. Please do not move your head." "I'm going to check your nose." "Say 'ah.'"	Letting the tongue rest on the floor of the mouth rather than protruding it actually improves visibility.
Weber	"Now I need to check your hearing. I'm going to put this tuning fork on your head. Tell me if it sounds the same in both ears or if it's louder in one ear."	
Rinne	"I'm going to put the tuning fork behind your ear. Can you hear this? Tell me when you can't hear it any longer." Once the patient can no longer hear it, move tuning fork anterior to ear and ask, "Can you hear it now?"	
Thyroid Auscultation of gland Palpation of gland	"Now I need to check your neck area." "I'm going to press lightly on your neck, so I'll need you to swallow. Would you like some water? Okay, let me get it. Please take a drink and hold it until I ask you to swallow."	The word "thyroid" may be considered medical terminology. Demonstrates empathy to offer water to help patient swallow more easily. If patient doesn't want water, don't insist.
Palpation of skin	"I need to check your skin."	Check for myxedema.
Hair brittleness	"I need to check your hair."	
Check for tremors	"Please hold out your hands like this and close your eyes."	Demonstrate how patient should hold hands.

Neurologic Exam

A complete neurologic exam is not possible during the CS exam because of its length; the parts that are appropriate will depend on the differential diagnosis.

- If a patient presents with symptoms consistent with cerebral vascular disease or subdural hematoma, focus the exam on detecting an upper motor neuron lesion. This could include cranial nerves, motor neurons, and light touch of all 4 extremities.

- If a patient with diabetes mellitus presents with symptoms of peripheral neuropathy, focus on testing the 4 sensory modalities—light touch, pain (using toothpicks on the CS), vibration, and position—and the deep tendon reflexes on both upper and lower limbs.

- Listen for a carotid bruit in the presence of symptoms of a transient ischemic episode (attack), i.e., TIA.

- Carpal tunnel syndrome is the most common entrapment neuropathy. Know the sensory distribution of the median nerve and the small muscles of the hand innervated by the nerve. Tapping the flexor retinaculum with a finger or reflex hammer will elicit dysesthesias in the sensory distribution of the median nerve (Tinel's sign).

Components of the Neurologic Exam

Not all components will be necessary.

Mental status

- Orientation (level of consciousness, orientation to person, place, and time)
- Concentration (spell "world" backward)
- Memory (remember 3 things); ask to repeat after a few minutes

Cranial nerves

- CN I: not tested
- CN II: vision (acuity, visual fields, PERRLA)
- CN III, IV, VI: extraocular movements
- CN V: sensation on face (all 3 areas) and motor component (clench your teeth)
- CN VII: close eyes tightly; smile; raise eyebrows
- CN VIII: hearing testing
- CN IX, X: look for symmetry of uvula
- CN XI: trapezius and sternocleidomastoid movement and power
- CN XII: protrude tongue

Upper limbs (compare one side to the other)

- Test tone and strength by passively flexing and extending
- Test biceps muscles and wrist extensors against resistance

Lower limbs (compare one side to the other)

- Test tone and strength by passively flexing and extending at the joints.
- Test flexors of the hip (iliopsoas) and dorsiflexors of the feet (tibialis anterior) against resistance.

(Continued)

Components of the Neurologic Exam (*Cont'd*)

Reflexes (not all are needed for every patient): biceps, triceps, brachioradialis, patellar, Achilles, Babinski

- **Biceps (C5, C6):** Patient's arm should be partially flexed at the elbow with palm down. Place your thumb or finger firmly on the biceps tendon. Strike with the reflex hammer so that the blow is aimed directly through your digit toward the biceps tendon.

- **Triceps (C6, C7):** Flex patient's arm at the elbow and pull it slightly across the chest. Strike the triceps tendon above the elbow.

- **Brachioradialis-Supinator Reflex (C5, C6):** Patient's hand should rest on the abdomen or the lap, with the forearm partly pronated. Strike the radius 1-2 inches above the wrist. Watch for flexion and supination.

- **Quadriceps-Knee Reflex (L2, L3, L4):** Briskly tap the patellar tendon below the patella. Note contraction of the quadriceps with extension at the knee. A hand on the patient's anterior thigh lets you feel this reflex. The quadriceps are the strongest muscles in the body so expect a forceful response.

- **Gastrocnemius-Ankle Reflex (primarily S1)**

  - If patient is sitting, dorsiflex the foot at the ankle. Strike the Achilles tendon. Watch and feel for plantar flexion.

  - If patient is lying down, flex one leg at both hip and knee and rotate it externally so that the lower leg rests across the opposite shin. Then, dorsiflex the foot at the ankle and strike the Achilles tendon.

- **Plantar Response (L5, S1) and the Babinski Response:** With an object such as the other end of a reflex hammer or the wooden end of an applicator stick, stroke the lateral aspect of the sole from the heel to the ball of the foot, curving medially across the ball. Use the lightest stimulus that will provoke a response. Note movements of the toes, normally flexion. Dorsiflexion of the big toe, often accompanied by fanning of the other toes, constitutes a Babinski response.

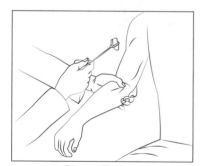

Biceps Reflex

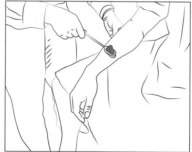

Brachioradialis Reflex

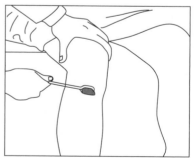

Patellar Reflex

Sensory

- Demonstrate sharp/dull
- Tell patient to close eyes
- Test sensory regions related to presenting complaint
- Repeat with light touch
- Test position sense using the big toe
- For vibration sense, test on the first metatarsal joint of each foot

Cerebellar

- Finger to nose
- Heel to shin
- Rapid alternating hand movements
- Gait: ask patient to walk across room

Specific Tests

Romberg sign (to assess the posterior columns, i.e., position sense, in a patient with unsteady gait/balance): Ask patient to stand with feet together. (Be ready to assist in case patient begins to fall.) First, test stability with patient's eyes open. If patient is steady with eyes open, repeat with eyes closed.

Kernig sign (when meningitis is suspected): With patient lying supine flex a knee, extend the leg on the thigh. A positive test is flexion of the neck as you extend the leg.

Brudzinski sign (when meningitis is suspected): If positive, gently flexing the neck results in flexion of both knees.

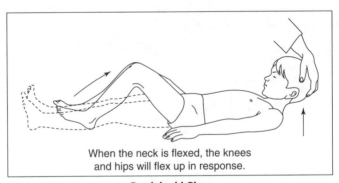

When the neck is flexed, the knees
and hips will flex up in response.

Brudzinski Sign

Suggested Phrasing for Neurologic Exam

Action	Suggested Phrasing	Comments
PERRLA	"I need to check your eyes."	
Funduscopic	"Now I need to shine the light so I can examine the back of your eyes. Thank you."	If patient resists, say, "I need to look at the blood vessels back there to make sure they're not damaged. It's extremely important for your safety."
Cranials **3, 4, 6**	"Follow my finger without moving your head."	
5	"I'm going to touch your face lightly. Tell me every time I do so."	Do for all 3 branches. Then say, "Now you may open your eyes."
7	"Close your eyes tightly and resist my trying to open them."	If any sentence is difficult for you to pronounce, just demonstrate the action and say, "Do this."
7	"Smile and show me your teeth." "Raise your eyebrows."	
8	"I'm going to rub my fingers next to your ear. Point to the side you hear it on. Now close your eyes."	
9, 10	"Open your mouth so I can see your throat."	
11	"Now shrug your shoulders." "Turn your face against my hand."	
12	"Now stick out your tongue."	
Upper limbs **Muscle testing**	"First I will check the tension in your muscles by moving them." "Now I will test your strength." (Remember "MRS": Muscles). "Make a muscle and resist me from pushing your arms down." "Extend your wrists and resist me from *— pull up* pushing them down."	Remember "MRS": Muscles
Reflexes **Sensory** **Light touch**	"I will tap on your arms for reflexes." (Reflexes) "Now I need to check your sense of touch." "Now I'm going to touch your hands lightly. Tell me if you feel it. Does it feel the same? Okay, now close your eyes."	Reflexes Sensation Repeat for 3 points on hand then say, "Okay, you may open your eyes now."
Sharp and dull	"Now I need to check your sharp and dull sensation. This is sharp. This is dull. Please close your eyes and tell me what you feel. Which is this? And this? How about this?"	Repeat for 3 points on hand. Then say, "Please open your eyes."

(Continued)

Suggested Phrasing for Neurologic Exam (*continued*)

Action	Suggested Phrasing	Comments
Lower extremities	"I need to check your leg strength. May I raise the sheet? Thank you."	
Muscle testing	"First I will check the tension in your muscles by moving them."	Test patella and Achilles.
	"Now I will test your strength."	
	"Extend your entire lower limb, resisting as I try to push down."	
	"Now move your foot toward your nose, resisting as I try to push down."	
Reflexes	"Now I'm going to tap on your legs."	Tap in 2 areas.
Babinski	"Now I will stroke the bottom of your feet."	
Sensory		
Light touch	"I'm going to touch your legs lightly. Tell me if you feel this. Please close your eyes and tell me every time you feel it."	Repeat for 3 points. "Please open your eyes."
Sharp and dull	"Now I need to check your responses to sharp and dull touch. This is sharp. This is dull. Please close your eyes. Which is this? How about this?"	Repeat for 3 points on feet. "Please open your eyes."
Vibration	"I'm placing this on your toe. Close your eyes. What do you feel? Please open your eyes."	
Position sense	"Now I'll be moving your toe. This is up, and this is down. Now tell me if it is up or down. Please close your eyes. You may open your eyes."	
Cerebellar		
Finger to nose	"Please touch your nose with your finger, then touch mine."	Hold up your own index finger to demonstrate.
Heel to shin	"Please do this. Do the same with your other leg."	
Gait	"Now I need to see how you walk. Let me pull out the footstool. May I help you step down? Please walk to the other side of the room and back. I'll stay with you."	Physically assisting the patient shows empathy.
Romberg	"Please stand with your feet together and close your eyes." (*demonstrate this*) "I will stand next to you to prevent you from falling. If you start to lose your balance, open your eyes."	Demonstrate action. Such phrases show empathy.
Kernig	"I need to uncover your leg. I'm going to bend your knee and then straighten it. Tell me if it hurts."	
Brudzinski	"I'm going to gently flex your neck and will stop if there is pain. Just relax while I do this."	

Pulmonary Exam

Do a pulmonary exam when there are complaints of cough, shortness of breath, wheezing, chest pain, and symptoms of upper respiratory infection. Do a thorough exam of the lungs whenever there are symptoms of pulmonary disease. Since you will be behind the patient at times and he won't be able to see what you are doing, it is important to let the patient know in advance before you do each step.

Inspection

- Examine for the presence of dyspnea or use of accessory muscles

Palpation

- Examine for chest wall tenderness
- Assess symmetrical expansion by placing hands posteriorly at level of 10th ribs
- Check tactile fremitus (say "99"); compare side-to-side; examine 6 regions posteriorly:
  - At lung apex
  - Adjacent to medial aspect of each scapula
  - At each lung base
- Then examine 4 regions anteriorly:
  - At lung apex
  - In both mid-axillary lines at midpoint of thorax

Percussion

It is critical to compare the right side to the left. Ask the patient to untie the gown.

- Lay your nondominant hand over the left lung apex; apply pressure and, using your dominant middle finger, tap on the middle finger of the nondominant hand (using a wrist hammering motion with your dominant wrist).
- Percuss the left lung apex, then immediately compare this percussion note (which is a hollow sound) to the percussion note of the right lung apex.
- Next, move to the mid-portion of the left lung and compare the note to that of the right.
- Finally, come down to the left lung base and compare the note to the right lung base. This way, both lungs have been done symmetrically.

Auscultation

Auscultation of the lungs is strongly recommended when there are primary pulmonary symptoms. Always compare side to side. Let the patient inhale/exhale before moving to the next area.

- Listen to the 6 posterior regions. Ask the patient to open her mouth and take deep, slow breaths in and out. Make sure you listen to a full inspiration and expiration in each region.
- Start with the left apex and compare it to the right.
- Move to the mid-portion of the left lung and compare it to that of the right.
- Finally, compare the left base to the right. Note any difference you hear on the left side compared to the right. (The patient may "fake" taking a deep breath when you listen to the right lung; if that happens, write "No breath sounds in right lung" in your Patient Note. This could happen with a pneumothorax case.)
- Examine 4 regions of the lungs anteriorly, comparing both sides.
- Now compare the left thorax lateral to the heart—lingual segments—with the right anterior thorax—middle lobe; perform fremitus, percussion, and auscultation.

Suggested Phrasing for Pulmonary Exam

Action	Suggested Phrasing	Comments
Posterior chest	"Please untie your gown. I need to check your lungs."	
Respiratory excursion	"I'm going to place my hands around your back. Please take a deep breath."	
Tactile fremitus	"Please say 99. Again."	Repeat at each level.
Percussion	"Now I'm going to tap on your chest/back."	Repeat at each level
Auscultation of lungs	"I need to listen to your lungs. Please take deep breaths in and out through your mouth."	Repeat at each level.
Anterior chest	"Please untie your gown."	
Tactile fremitus	"Please say 99. Again."	Repeat at each level.
Percussion	"Now I'm going to tap on your chest."	
Auscultation of lungs	"Let me listen to your lungs. Please breathe in and out through your mouth. Thank you."	

A change in the color (cyanosis, pallor) or shape of nails/digits can be a clue for serious systemic or chronic disease. Be sure to inspect them when doing a complete respiratory or cardiovascular examination.

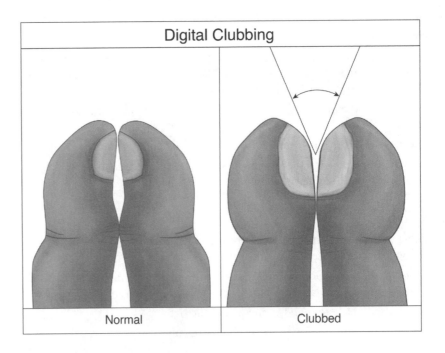

Digital Clubbing

Normal   Clubbed

Cardiovascular Exam

Do a cardiovascular exam when there are complaints of chest pain, palpitations, shortness of breath, loss of consciousness, or pedal edema.

- Examine external jugular vein. Place the table at a 30° angle. Ask the patient to turn his head slightly to the left. Shine a light source obliquely over the area of the external jugular vein on the right side of the patient's neck.

- Ask the patient to lower the upper edge of the gown to the level of the bra/breasts. Listen over the second left intercostal space to the pulmonic valve and then to the aortic valve over the second right intercostal space.

- Ask female patients to assist by moving the gown down to the waist. Then have them lift their breast slightly while you say, "I am looking for your heartbeat and will touch the area to identify where the beat is located."

- Auscultate the heart beginning at the apical impulse (mitral valve). Move your stethoscope horizontally to the left parasternal line (tricuspid valve). Readjust the gown to where it was located. Auscultate while patient is sitting and again lying down at 30°.

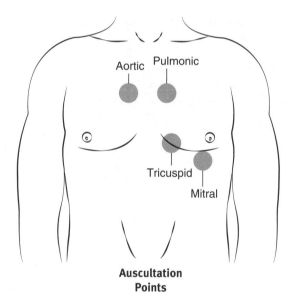

Auscultation Points

- Examine peripheral pulses
  - If appropriate, listen for a carotid bruit at the bifurcation of both common carotid arteries (located anterior to sternocleidomastoid on a horizontal line drawn from the thyroid notch). Do not palpate the bifurcation site because one may activate a baroreceptor within the carotid sinus, which is located superior to the bifurcation in the wall of the internal carotid artery and cause bradycardia or a vasovagal response.

  - When appropriate, examine the peripheral pulses in the lower limbs: start with posterior tibial, and dorsalis pedis. If these are not palpable then move proximally to the popliteal then femoral arteries.

  - Palpate pulses distal to an acute injury. For example, if an 18-year-old boy fell off his scooter and hurt his left elbow, palpate the radial and ulnar arteries.

Suggested Phrasing for Cardiovascular Exam

Action	Suggested Phrasing	Comments
Sitting up		
Carotid bruit	"I need to listen to your neck sounds. Breathe in and out 3 times, then hold your breath."	
Palpation of pulses	"I'm going to check your pulses."	
Edema	"I'm going to check your legs for swelling."	
Inspection and palpation of apical impulse	"I need to examine your heartbeat."	For women, you may need to ask, "Please lift your breast. Thank you."
Auscultation of heart	"I need to listen to your heart."	Leave gown untied.
Lying down		
Jugular venous distention	"Please look to the left. I need to take a look at your neck."	Adjust table for JVD and pull out extension.
Costochondral tenderness	"Now I need to press on your chest. Any pain?"	Maintain eye contact.
Epigastric tenderness	"Now I need to press on your stomach area."	

Abdominal Exam

Do an abdominal exam when there are complaints of the following:

- Abdominal pain, diarrhea, constipation
- Nausea, vomiting
- Weight loss or decreased appetite
- Hematochezia, hematemesis
- Jaundice
- UTI symptoms/hematuria
- Pelvic pain
- Pregnancy
- Abnormal vaginal bleeding
- Sexual dysfunction

Inspection

- Properly drape the patient by lifting the gown to just above the costal margins; move the sheet to above the inguinal ligaments. Inspect for distension, scars, rashes, bruises, or any other abnormality; tell the patient that you are inspecting the skin.

Auscultation

- Auscultate for bowel sounds **prior** to percussion and palpation. Listen for 3 seconds in each of the 4 quadrants.
- If you are considering partial rupture of an abdominal aortic aneurysm, listen for a bruit over the surface projection of the abdominal aorta.

Percussion

- Tap twice over each of the 4 quadrants.
- To evaluate for the presence of ascites, percuss starting at the umbilicus moving toward the flanks.
- If indicated, evaluate for the presence of an enlarged liver. The percussed span of the liver in the right mid-clavicular line correlates with the true size of the liver.
- Percuss the superior border by moving inferiorly from the resonance of normal lung to dullness.
- Then percuss the inferior border by moving superiorly from abdominal tympany to dullness.
- Normal liver span is 8-12 cm; taller women and men have longer spans.
  - During the Step 2 CS exam, it is impossible to accurately measure the span of the liver in women because of the presence of the bra.
  - For women, percuss the inferior border only.

Palpation

- Gently palpate the abdomen in all 4 quadrants.
  - Watch the patient's face for any indication of discomfort or pain.
  - Do not use excessive force, as it may harm the SP.
- Note any areas with rebound tenderness.
- If indicated, evaluate for the presence of an enlarged spleen.
  - The normal spleen is not palpable.
  - Do not use excessive force.

Consider the following **special maneuvers** while performing an abdominal exam (note that for some of these maneuvers, there may be more than one way to perform)

- **CVA tenderness** (common during episodes of acute pyelonephritis)
  - Lightly tap the costovertebral angle.
  - If tenderness is present, the test is positive.

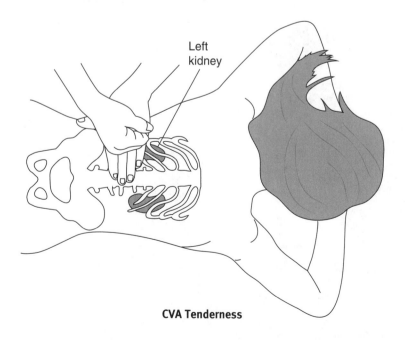

Left kidney

CVA Tenderness

- **Psoas sign**
  - Place your hand above the patient's right knee and ask patient to raise the thigh against resistance.
  - If abdominal pain in the right lower quadrant is increased, the test is positive.
- **Obturator sign**
  - Place one hand on the patient's ankle and the other hand on the knee.
  - Internally rotate the hip by moving the ankle externally (this pushes the obturator muscle to stretch).
  - If there is pain, an inflamed appendix is located retrocecally or in the pelvic area.

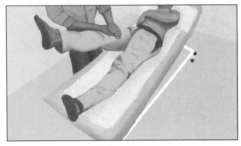 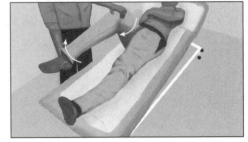

Psoas Sign	**Obturator Sign**

- **Rebound tenderness**
  - Press firmly on patient's abdomen and release quickly.
  - Increased pain on quick withdrawal suggests peritoneal irritation.
- **Rovsing's sign**
  - Palpate left lower quadrant
  - If pain is increased in the right lower quadrant, the test is positive.
- **Murphy's sign**
  - Palpate inferior to the right costal margin.
  - If there is cessation of respiration during deep inspiration, the test is positive.

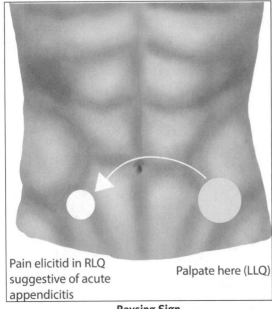

Pain elicitid in RLQ suggestive of acute appendicitis

Palpate here (LLQ)

Rovsing Sign

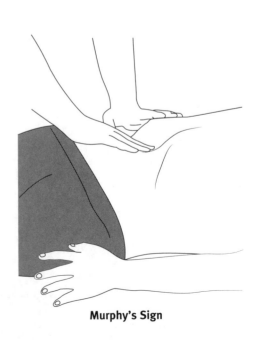

Murphy's Sign

Suggested Phrasing for Abdominal Exam

Action	Suggested Phrasing	Comments
Inspection	"Let me take a look at your abdomen."	If you notice any scars or abnormalities, ask about them.
Auscultation	"Now I need to listen to your abdomen."	Let the patient know that your stethoscope may be cold.
Light palpation	"I need to press lightly on your abdomen."	Examine painful areas last.
Percussion	"I need to tap on your abdomen."	
Rebound tenderness	"Now I need to press in on your abdomen. Tell me if it hurts more when I press in or let go."	
CVA tenderness	"I'm going to gently tap on your back. Let me know if it hurts."	
Special test for cholecystitis Murphy's sign	"I need to press in on your abdomen. Please take a deep breath and let me know if it hurts."	

Musculoskeletal Exam

Musculoskeletal pain is a common reason Americans visit physicians. Symptoms are usually located in one region or one joint. Lumbosacral strain and intervertebral disc protrusion or herniation—in either cervical or lumbar regions—are common. Straight-leg raising test will exacerbate pain if there is sensory root compression. Examine the sacroiliac joints and gait when evaluating a patient with low back pain.

Do a musculoskeletal exam when there are complaints of:

- Joint pain
- Extremity pain
- An acute injury
- Decreased range of motion
- Weakness or fatigue
- Any rheumatology case

To assess the presence of the most common disc herniations or protrusions, use the following guidelines.

DISC /ROOT	REFLEX	MUSCLE/SENSATION
C6-C7 C7	Triceps	Wrist drop/extensors; second & third fingers
L4-L5 L5	Patellar	Foot drop/tibialis anterior; great toe
L5-S1 S1	Achilles	Gastrocnemius; lateral foot

- Always compare the affected side to the normal one
- Palpate the joint distal and proximal to the complaint joint
- Inspect the joint or region for erythema or swelling; palpate for warmth and tenderness. Performing an active range of motion with the patient facilitates the exam.

Because it is often challenging to identify the exact location of an abnormality, shoulder and neck are examined as one region, regardless of where the pain is located. After testing the active range of motion of shoulder joints, test internal and external rotation passively.

- Elbow region is examined for the presence of epicondylitis, when appropriate
- Wrist/hand is evaluated for carpal tunnel syndrome (see figure below)
  - Tinel: tap the wrist at the flexor retinaculum (over the median nerve)
  - Phalen: patient places dorsum of hands together facing downward
- Hip joints are examined passively to more accurately test range of motion (internal rotation, external rotation, flexion, and extension if concerned that the patient has arthritis of the hip (patient must lie on abdomen, face down, or stand/extend the leg backward)
- Knee joints: anterior and posterior drawer, medial and lateral collateral ligaments, McMurray's
- Ankle joints and feet are examined as one region, actively and passively (see figure below).
  - Palpate the plantar fascia to assess for the presence of plantar fasciitis; note the increase in tenderness at the point the fascia inserts on the calcaneus
  - If appropriate, perform a limited neurologic examination of the affected region
  - Assess vascular status (pulses) in the affected region. Musculoskeletal and neurologic exams have areas of similarity.

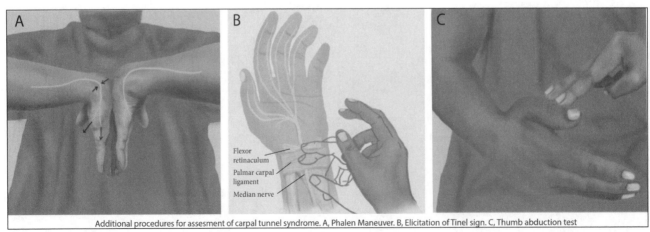

Additional procedures for assesment of carpal tunnel syndrome. A, Phalen Maneuver. B, Elicitation of Tinel sign. C, Thumb abduction test

Carpal Tunnel Maneuvers

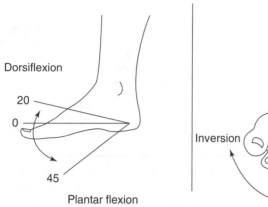 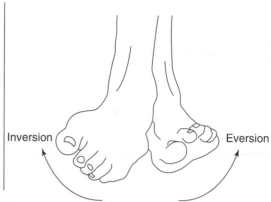

Range of Motion of Ankles

Suggested Phrasing for Musculoskeletal Exam

Action	Suggested Phrasing	Comments
Always let the patient know beforehand when you're going to untie, raise, or lower the gown. Tie the gown when your examination is complete.		
Wrist pain Inspection	"Let me take a look at your wrist and other joints."	Paraphrasing what the patient has told you shows care and concern.
Palpation	"I know you have pain on this side, so let me start with the normal side first. Now let me check this side."	
Active range of movement	"Now I need to see how your joints are moving. Let me start with the one that doesn't hurt."	
Passive range of movement	"I will now gently move your joints."	
Muscle testing for UE	"Do this. Don't let me push in. Don't let me push out. Do this. Don't let me push up. Don't let me push down. Do this. Don't let me squeeze your fingers together. Do this. Squeeze my fingers as hard as you can."	Don't say "ouch!" if the patient squeezes too hard.
Reflexes for UE	"Now I need to tap on your arm."	Tap in 3 areas on each hand.
Sensory	"Now I'll check your sensation."	
Light touch	"I need to touch your hands lightly. Tell me if you feel this. Please close your eyes. Do you feel this? How about this? Does it feel the same?"	Repeat for 3 points on hand. "Please open your eyes now."
Sharp and dull	"Now I'll check your sharp and dull touch. This is sharp. This is dull. Okay, please close your eyes. Which is this? Which is this?"	Repeat for 3 points on hand. "You may open your eyes now."
Carpal tunnel evaluation		
Tinel	"I need to tap on your wrists. Let me start with the one that doesn't hurt."	
Phalen	"Do this. Let me know if it hurts."	Demonstrate action.

Shoulder pain
  Inspection
  Palpation
	"Let me take a look at your shoulder and other joints."
	"I know you said it hurts, so I'll start with the other one. I need to untie your gown. Okay, now I'm going to press on your neck. Any pain? Now your shoulder blade [or] Now here. Any pain? Now let me do the same on the other side. Let me tie your gown back."	

Range of movement	"I need to check on your shoulder movement. With the hand that doesn't hurt, do this. This. This. Now with the other hand, go only as far as you can. Do this. Do this. This. Thank you."	Repeat for other shoulder.

UE = upper extremity; LE = lower extremity

(Continued)

Suggested Phrasing for Musculoskeletal Exam (*continued*)

Action	Suggested Phrasing	Comments
Muscle testing for UE	"I need to check your arm strength. Do this. Don't let me push in. Don't let me push out. Do this. Don't let me push up. Do this. Don't let me push down. Don't let me squeeze your fingers together. Do this. Squeeze my fingers as hard as you can."	
Reflexes for UE	"Now I need to tap on your arms."	Repeat for 3 areas.
Sensory for UE		
Light touch	"I need to check your sensation. May I pull up your sleeves? Thank you. Now I'm going to touch your hands lightly. Do you feel this? Please close your eyes. Do you feel this? And this? Does it feel the same? Do you feel this? This? Does it feel the same?"	Besides the 3 points on hand, check deltoid area. Repeat for 4 points. "Please open your eyes."
Sharp and dull	"Now let's check sharp and dull. This is sharp. This is dull. Which is this? This?"	Repeat for 4 points. "Please open your eyes."
Lower back pain		
Inspection	"Let me take a look at your other joints."	
Palpation	"I need to press on your back. Now I'm going to press over here. May I untie your gown?"	
Muscle testing for LE	"I need to check your leg strength. Push out. Pull back. Push on the gas [or] Push down. Pull up."	
Reflexes	"Now I'll tap on your legs."	
Sensory for LE		
Light touch	"I need to check your sensation. I'm going to touch your legs lightly. Do you feel this? Now please close your eyes. Do you feel this? This? Does it feel the same?"	Repeat for 4 points. "Open your eyes."
Sharp and dull	"Now I need to check your sharp and dull touch. This is sharp. This is dull. Okay, please close your eyes. Which is this? This?"	Repeat for 4 points. "Open your eyes."
Babinski	"Now I need to tickle your feet [or] I need to scratch your feet."	
Gait	"I need to see how you walk. Let me pull out the footstool. May I help you down? Please walk to the other side of the room and back. I'll be nearby."	
Range of motion	"Please bend down and try to touch your toes. Now twist from side to side [or] Do this. Now, lean back."	Demonstrate twisting.
Knee pain		
Inspection	"Let me check your knees."	
Palpation	"I know you said this knee hurts, so I'll start with the other one. Let me lift the sheet so I can press on your knee."	
Range of motion	"Let's see how your leg moves."	
Muscle testing for LE	"Let's check your leg strength. Push out. Pull back. Push on the gas [or] Push down. Pull up."	
Reflexes	"Now I need to tap on your legs."	
Sensory for LE		
Light tough	"I need to check your sensation. I'm going to touch your feet lightly. Do you feel this? Please close your eyes. Can you feel this? How about this? Is it the same? Do you feel this? This? Is it the same?"	Repeat for 4 points. "You can open your eyes now."
Sharp and dull	"Now let's check your sense of sharp and dull. This is sharp. This is dull. Okay, please close your eyes. Which is this? This?"	Repeat for 4 points. "Please open your eyes."
Pulses	"I need to check your pulses."	
Knee joint effusion	"Let's see if you have any swelling. Okay, now the other knee."	
Anterior/posterior drawer sign	"I need to push and pull on your knee. Okay, now the other one."	
McMurray	"I'm going to push down on your knee and move your foot. Okay, now the other knee."	
Collateral strain	"I need to push on your knee. Now the other one."	

Psychiatry Mental Status Exam

Perform the psychiatric mental status exam when the history provided by the standardized patient supports a likely psychiatric diagnosis.

General Appearance

Assess the patient's grooming, facial expressions, level of eye contact, body movement, and attitude toward physician.

- Unkempt appearance and poor eye contact can be seen in depression or psychosis
- Provocative dressing can be seen in bipolar disorder
- Psychomotor retardation can be seen in depression or schizophrenia
- Psychomotor agitation can be seen in mania or anxiety

Speech

Assess the quantity, quality, volume, and rate of speech.

- Rapid, pressured speech with flight of ideas with connections can be seen in mania
- Speech diminished in both quantity and content with looseness of associations can be seen in schizophrenia
- Speech slower and diminished in quantity can also be seen in depression
- Rapid speech can be seen with anxiety

Orientation

Assess if the patient is oriented to person, place and time. Ask the patient to state their full name. Ask what city they are in. Ask the current year and month or day of the week.

Recent Memory

Assess if the patient can immediately repeat 3 objects and then recall them after several minutes. Say, "Please repeat the following 3 objects: cat, apple, and table. Please remember them so that you can repeat them again when I ask you."

Attention and Concentration

Assess by asking the patient to spell the word "world" backward or to subtract serial sevens from 100 (however, take into account that subtracting serial sevens from 100 may be difficult for someone with limited math skills).

Mood

Mood is a subjective internal feeling reported by the patient. Ask, "How have you felt during the past few weeks?" Common adjectives used to describe mood include depressed, anxious, angry, hopeless, irritable, happy, and euphoric.

Affect

Affect is an objective observation by the physician. It can be consistent with mood or inappropriate based on the details of the encounter (e.g., a patient with schizophrenia may laugh or respond with a flat, unemotional response during a discussion about death).

Note

- **Anxiety** can cause immediate and recent memory deficits.

- **Depression** can cause pseudo-dementia.

Hallucinations

Hallucinations are perceptual disturbances that can be auditory, visual, tactile, olfactory, gustatory or visceral. Look for auditory hallucinations in schizophrenia. You may observe the standardized patient talking to himself when you enter the room. Look for visual hallucinations in alcohol withdrawal and drug abuse cases. Ask:

- "Do you see things that others don't?"
- "Do you hear voices when you are alone?"
- "Do you obey the commands of these voices or ignore what they tell you to do?"
- "Do you feel, smell or taste things that are not really there?"

Delusions

Delusions are fixed, false beliefs inconsistent with reality. Ask:

- "Do people think you have an unrealistic view of yourself or life in general?"
- "Do you think you have special powers or abilities?"
- "Have others commented that your thoughts are strange?"
- "Do you think people want to harm you?"
- "Do you think people want to put ideas in your head or steal your thoughts?"
- "Do you think people are jealous of you and want everything that you have?"
- "Do you think people are talking behind your back or stealing from you?"

Delusions can be congruent with mood, such as having delusions of grandeur with the elated mood seen in mania. Mood-incongruent delusions support a diagnosis of schizophrenia.

Suicide

Suicide risk will be increased when there is a (1) definite plan, (2) previous attempt that failed, and (3) family history of suicide in a first-degree relative. Ask if the patient wants to harm or kill him or herself.

Homicide

Ask if the patient wants to harm or kill others.

Insight

Assess the patient's understanding of her own feelings and illnesses. Ask what she attributes her symptoms to and the impact on her life.

A lack of ability to understand one's feelings and potential illness is seen in both schizophrenia and manic phases of bipolar disorder.

Judgment

Assess the patient's ability to understand the consequences of her actions. Present a hypothetical scenario and ask the standardized patient what she would do under those circumstances. Examples include walking into a room and seeing a fire burning in a garbage can or seeing a stamped envelope on the sidewalk.

Bizarre responses not similar to putting out the fire and mailing the letter represent impaired judgment and are consistent with psychosis.

Immediately after each patient encounter in Step 2 CS, you will be asked to type (on a computer) a Patient Note similar to the medical record you would compose after seeing a patient in a clinic, office, or emergency department.

The Patient Note is an important component of the ICE score and the only component of the CS exam graded by a physician. You will be graded using a global rating scale and not a specific checklist. Your note must therefore reflect an intelligent logical approach to patient care and differential diagnosis.

PATIENT NOTE LOGISTICS

We encourage you to become familiar with the Orientation and Practice Materials for Step 2 CS, including Patient Note interactive simulations and samples of Patient Notes that are available at **usmle.org**. Your Patient Note practice should be conducted in the format available on that web page, which is the same format that will be used on the day of your exam.

You will be required to type all your Patient Notes. Stay within the space allotted for each section. There are characters as well as line limits for each field on the Patient Note screen as follows:

- **History:** 950 characters, 15 lines
- **Physical Examination:** 950 characters, 15 lines
- **Diagnosis:** 100 characters for each diagnosis
- **History Findings and Physical Examination Findings:** 100 characters per field
- **Diagnostic Studies:** 100 characters per study recommendation

You may add rows to History Supporting Findings, Physical Examination Supporting Findings, and Diagnostic Studies sections (up to 8 rows each). The Patient Note screen that appears during the actual exam will have a status bar for both history and physical examination, indicating how many characters have been used.

A blank sheet of paper is provided for writing brief notes during the actual USMLE encounters. These notes are not read and therefore not factored into your overall Patient Note performances.

PATIENT NOTE ORGANIZATION

To the best of your ability, use correct grammar and sentence structure. An occasional misspelled word—as long as it does not change the meaning of that word—could be acceptable. Practice spelling words that are commonly misspelled—*pneumonia, abscess, inflammation,* and *ischemia*—and any other common medical terms that give you difficulty.

A good Patient Note, in particular good history and physical, will involve typing what you **asked of** the patient, what **exam** you did, and what you have **observed during encounters**.

Note

If no physical exam is performed (as in a phone case), leave the physical exam section blank.

There are 4 components to every Patient Note:

- History
- Physical Examination
- Differential Diagnosis (1–3 rows)
- Diagnostic Workup (1–8 rows)

CLINICAL SKILLS EVALUATION
PATIENT NOTE

HISTORY: Describe the history you just obtained from this patient. Include only information (pertinent positives and negatives) relevant to this patient's problem(s).

PHYSICAL EXAMINATION: Describe any positive and negative findings relevant to this patient's problem(s). Be careful to include *only* those parts of examination you performed in *this* encounter.

DATA INTERPRETATION: *Based on what you have learned from the history and physical examination*, list up to 3 diagnoses that might explain this patient's complaint(s). List your diagnoses from most to least likely. For some cases, fewer than 3 diagnoses will be appropriate. Then, enter the positive or negative findings from the history and the physical examination (if present) that support each diagnosis. Lastly, list initial *diagnostic* studies (if any) you would order for each listed diagnosis (e.g. restricted physical exam maneuvers, laboratory tests, imaging, ECG, etc.).

DIAGNOSIS #1:

HISTORY FINDING(S)	PHYSICAL EXAM FINDING(S)

(+) Click to add row(s)

DIAGNOSIS #2:

HISTORY FINDING(S)	PHYSICAL EXAM FINDING(S)

(+) Click to add row(s)

DIAGNOSIS #3:

HISTORY FINDING(S)	PHYSICAL EXAM FINDING(S)

(+) Click to add row(s)

DIAGNOSTIC STUDIES

(+) Click to add row(s)

History

The history section contains all of the information subjectively given to you by patients. This includes the "story" about their chief complaint (HPI), all of the **pertinent positives/negatives** from the ROS, PMH, meds, allergies, and **pertinent social/family history**.

- Focus sharply on HPI and include pertinent positives and negatives
- Consider and document only relevant components of PMH
- To get a point for the CC, 3 components are needed: age, gender, complaint (e.g. 68 yo M c/o chest pain)

Note

Common abbreviations can be used to save time and space in your Patient Note. See the **Appendix** for an extensive list of potential abbreviations.

History of Present Illness (HPI) and Past Medical History (PMH):

The history section should include all information that you have been collecting during the encounters using the mnemonics. **PMH** includes all pertinent information with regards to the individual patient, their chief complaint, and your differential diagnosis. It includes serious illnesses/significant hospitalizations/surgeries, medications, allergies, and pertinent social/family history. See chapter 3 for details on history taking.

When typing the history component of your Patient Note, to save time and characters, consider using phrases rather than sentences:

- *64 y/o woman c/o substernal chest pain*
- *8/10 in intensity, heavy, crushing, constant pain*
- *Started 1 hour ago while watching TV*
- *Radiates to L arm and jaw*
- *Nothing makes it better. Worse with exertion*
- *(+) SOB, diaphoresis*
- *(–) syncope, fever, cough, palpitations, leg swelling*
- *No previous episodes*
- *No Rx or OTC meds, NKDA*
- *Denies hx of htn, dm, or high cholesterol*
- *(+) smoker (30 pack years), denies ETOH and drugs*
- *No family hx of heart disease*

For Past Medical History and Social History (PMHx/PSHx), "*not relevant*" is acceptable and requires no further detail.

Physical Examination

For the physical examination, start by listing the vitals (given on doorway information) and the general appearance. Record the focused physical examination that you performed, including both positive and negative findings.

- First, familiarize yourself with the normal exams of each tested systems.
- Then, think about how you would document an abnormality that may be present.

When typing your Patient Note, do not type components of the history and physical that you did not conduct. In cases where the patient is not present—phone case or surrogate—leave the physical exam section blank. Read carefully your doorway information; you will be given clear instructions on parts that you are not expected to do.

Physicians grading your notes are more concerned with your ability to communicate your objective physical findings than with your format or punctuation. Write phrases rather than sentences.

When considering how to take notes, follow this sample for general headings:

GA: general appearance

VS: vital signs

Chest or **Lungs:** chest

ABD or **Abd:** abdomen

HEENT: head, eyes, ears, nose, throat

Neuro: neurologic exam

CV: cardiovascular

UE & LE: upper extremity and lower extremity

Vital Signs

Vital signs (given on doorway information) should be noted on every Patient Note. If a patient's chief complaint is cough, and you noted on the doorway information that there was fever, **make sure to record or interpret** the fever (i.e., febrile) on your Note. That would be a pertinent vital sign most likely supporting your differential diagnosis.

If all vital signs are normal, you could use the abbreviation **WNL** (within normal limits). If only one vital sign is abnormal, you could state **VS: WNL except BP 150/100.**

In the presence of fever, respirations 30/min, pulse 120/min, and blood pressure 90/60 mm Hg, these would all be pertinent vital signs and should be recorded in the beginning of your physical examination component. For example:

- VS–90/60, p 120, RR 30, afebrile
- Vitals–120/80, p 86
- Vital signs–normal or VS WNL
- VS–T 40, BP 120/70, p 84
- Vitals normal except BP 180/90

Height and weight should be noted if relevant to the case; that would include a general physical or periodic health exam, pre-employment physical, life insurance, or any other time you think it may be relevant. For example:

- Wt–100 kg
- Weight 155 lbs; height 5 ft 2 inches

General Appearance (GA)

This is the place to describe the patient you saw sitting in front of you as you began your physical exam. Comment on any unusual behavior observed. It's fine if you have some components of psychiatric or mental status here in particular if your differential diagnoses are psychiatric. Some examples:

- GA: NAD (no acute distress)
- GA: in [mild/moderate/severe] distress from [pain/SOB]
- GA: no distress, A&O x3 (alert and oriented times 3)
- GA: pt is pacing the room in [pain/anger/rage]
- GA: dirty, torn clothes; smells of beer (or other body odor)
- GA: quiet, flat affect; will not make eye contact
- GA: track marks on arms, multiple bruises

Skin

Skin could be treated as a system on its own. Describe the anatomic location of any encountered color changes, tenderness, warmth, as well as the pattern of any flat/raised lesions as precisely as possible. Some examples:

- Skin: multiple blue/red macules on upper and lower ext in sun-exposed areas. Warm & tender. No streaks.
- Skin: jaundice (or Skin: yellow powder on face)
- Skin: [track/needle] marks on both arms

HEENT

While typing the note for each organ system you can follow the same outline that you are already familiar with from the physical examination section.(Inspection, Palpation, etc.). There is no need to type subheadings for eyes, ears, etc. The abbreviation HEENT stands for:

Head

Eye

Ear

Nose

Throat

A normal **HEENT** is given below:

HEENT: normocephalic/atraumatic (NC/AT), nontender. PERRLA. Fundi–red reflex intact, EOMI. Fundoscopy NL. No papilledema. Vison WNL. No visual defect. TMs, pharynx–WNL. Nasal turbinates not congested, no nasal discharge. No tonsilar enlargements, erythema, exudates, vesicular lesions. Neck supple. Lymph nodes NL, (or no LAD), thyroid not enlarged.

If abnormalities are found, be as specific as possible in describing them. For example:

- HEENT: tender, pre-auricular node and pinna, (-) redness,(-) swelling
- Head: deformity, tender with epistaxis from right nostril
- Head: b/l tenderness [maxillary sinus, cheek]
- Head: fine, thin hair. No exophthalmos [diaphoretic, sweating], no thyroid enlargement. [Tenderness, deformity, crepitus] to [nose, cheek, maxilla, jaw, zygoma, orbit, forehead]

Further examples of **HEENT** note-writing:

- PERRL: (pupils equal, round, reactive to light)
- PERRLA: (the "A" stands for "and accommodation")
- PERRLA: sclera clear, EOMI (extraocular movement intact). Extraocular muscles intact except [R 6th nerve palsy, R lateral gaze deficit].
- Visual fields intact, or R [temporal, nasal] visual field deficit
- Visual acuity: VA–20/20 OU (OU = both eyes, OS = left eye, OD = right eye). VA: 20/200 R eye, counting fingers 5 ft L eye.
- Visual acuity: L eye light perception only, OD–20/200. Fundi: flat (no papilledema), or Fundi: Not visualized, or Fundi–NL red reflex.

For nose, be as specific as possible:

No nasal discharge and/or good air entry b/l, or b/l thick yellow discharge, or nasal septum [intact/perforated]

For ears:

- *Pinna NL. TM WNL b/l (tympanic membrane normal bilaterally)*
- *R TM red bulging, L NL. (Right tympanic membrane is red and bulging, L tympanic membrane is normal)*
- *TMs both with [perforation/holes] b/l*

For throat:

- *Pharynx [clear, red, with exudates, NL]*

Teeth

- *[Dentition/Teeth], [poor/normal]*

Thyroid

- *Thyroid: [nontender/tender], [normal size/enlarged]. No nodules.*
- *Nontender, NL size, no nodules, trachea in midline; or Tender, enlarged, trachea shifted L*

Lymph nodes

You may examine a patient for cervical, axillary, and femoral triangle (inguinal) lymph nodes.

- *Lymph nodes: not swollen or tender - or no LAD*
- *Hard, tender supraclavicular lymph node*
- *Diffuse lymphadenopathy (seen with mononucleosis)*

You may also list the particular nodes that are swollen and tender, such as the following: [submandibular, submental, preauricular, postauricular, anterior cervical, posterior cervical, supraclavicular, subclavicular] adenopathy.

Chest/lungs

Remember to do a complete chest exam (inspection, palpation, respiratory excursion, tactile fremitus, percussion, and auscultation) and document all your findings. Again, document *everything* you do so you can maximize your score.

Normal chest exam:

- *Chest appears NL, nontender, NL resp, excursion, fremitus, percussion NL and equal b/l. Lungs clear to auscultation bilaterally; CTA b/l.*
- *Chest without deformity, skin WNL. Lungs clear to A&P b/l (A&P means "auscultation and percussion").*

Abnormal chest exam:

- *Inspection: Increase AP diameter, or pursed-lip breathing, or chest with deformity or [ecchymoses/bruise] R flank, or thoracotomy scar*
- *Palpation: Tenderness on [R lat 8th rib, L CVA, lumbar spine, R costochondral margin]. Be as specific as possible about the area of tenderness.*
- *Respiratory excursion: Poor respiratory excursion or paradoxical chest wall excursion*
- *Fremitus: [increased/decreased] fremitus [R/L] [base/midlung field/apex]*
- *Percussion: [dull/hyperresonant] percussion [R/L] [base/midfield/apex]*
- *Auscultation: [decreased/absent] breath sounds [L/R]. Or you may have heard abnormal sounds: [wheeze, rhonchi, rub, rales] [L/R] [base/midlung/apex]*

Cardiovascular

Normal cardiovascular exam:

within normal limits

Note

An irregularly irregular heart rhythm is often atrial fibrillation.

- *Regular rate & rhythm (RRR); apical impulse not displaced(PMI); S1, S2-WNL; no rub/gallop/murmur (MRG); no JVD, clubbing, or edema. No carotid artery bruits. Peripheral arterial pulses palpable in lower limbs.*

For the normal person, you could write **"No JVD"** or **"JVP NL"**; either notation is correct.

In fact, you could also write **"CV : S1, S2 WNL, RRR, no RMG."**

If abnormalities are found on the cardiovascular exam, be as specific as possible. Most SPs will have expectedly a normal CV exam.

For pulse:

[R/L] [radial/brachial/femoral/popliteal/DP/PT] pulse [absent/decreased/NL/bounding]

For point of maximal impulse (PMI):

PMI displaced

If you felt the apex, you can describe its location, e.g., PMI at anterior axillary line, 8th rib.

For heart rate and rhythm, the grading scale for murmur is as follows:

- 1/6 = faintest murmur
- 2/6 = soft murmur
- 3/6 = loud murmur
- 4/6 = very loud murmur with palpable thrill when you check PMI
- 5/6 = heard with stethoscope partly off the chest
- 6/6 = heard with stethoscope off the chest

[**RRR, irregular irregularly rhythm**] + **gallop rhythm** (Write this when you hear an S3 or S4 heart sound.)

[**1/6, 2/6, 3/6, 4/6**] [**diastolic/systolic**] **murmur** is the basic notation for murmur. A murmur can be pansystolic, early, or late.

Abdomen

Document the parts of physical examination that you have conducted: inspection, auscultation, percussion, and palpation.

Normal abdomen exam:

ABD: symmetric nl appearance, BS present, no bruits heard, liver span in right MCL = 10cm; spleen not palpable; no abd. mass. No tenderness.

Document all additional tests performed even if they are normal:

Murphy's sign: absent; no CVA tenderness; no flank dullness; negative Psoas and Obturator, Rovsing's and rebound

Accurately describe abnormalities:

- *Skin: record scars or other changes indicating correct anatomical delimitation*
- *Palpation: note location of direct or rebound tenderness by region or quadrant; indicate anatomical location of tests performed in the abdomen if they are positive*

Bowel sounds will always be present. Record with accuracy what **is present**, not what **should be present**.

Neurological

Think about the entire neurological exam and write down the parts that you have performed. If abnormalities are found, be as specific as possible in describing them.

Complete normal neurologic exam:

Neuro: A&O×3. CN 2 - 12 NL. Sensation to light touch, position sense and vibration sense intact all 4 ext. on lower ext NL B/L. Motor 5/5, DTR 2/4, B/L all 4 ext. Gait–WNL. No Kernig or Brudzinski. Neck supple. Straight leg raise negative B/L. Romberg negative. Coordination intact. No dysmetria or dysdiadochokinesia. Babinski–nl B/L.

For mental status abnormalities, if the patient knows only her name but not the place or date:

A & O x 1 (or Alert and oriented to person only)

For cranial nerves, you can interpret the physical finding or just describe it:

Pt points tongue out to L = L 12th nerve palsy

Entire R side of face is weak, pt cannot close R eye = R peripheral 7th CN lesion

For sensation, describe where the patient is experiencing numbness. Sensations described/tested are sharp, dull, vibration and position sense.

- *[Decreased/No] light touch below knee B/L; no position sense L toe, R lower ext. WNL*
- *Numbness R ulnar nerve distribution (Numb 5th digit R hand.)*

Motor

Motor function is traditionally graded on a 5-point scale.

0/5	flaccid
1/5	just a flicker of movement
2/5	so weak that the patient cannot overcome gravity
3/5	can overcome gravity
4/5	somewhat weak
5/5	normal

- *Motor: 3/5 RUE, other ext NL describes someone with a weak R arm and the other 3 extremities normal.*

You may also use regular language to describe the degree of weakness. For instance:

- *Motor: [Mild/Moderate/Severe] weakness RUE*
- *Motor: Pt with [dense paralysis/0/5] entire R side of body, L side WNL*

Reflexes

Reflexes are traditionally graded on a 4-point scale.

0/4	no reflex
1/4	decreased
2/4	normal
3/4	somewhat hyperreflexic
4/4	clonus (very hyperreflexic)

- *DTR: 1/4 brachial B/L (decreased reflex brachial DTR both sides)*
- *DTR: R brachial & patella 4/4, L 2/4 (patient who is hyperreflexic on R side of the body)*

Gait

- *Gait: ataxic if unsteady or patient unable to walk*
- *Romberg: positive if patient cannot perform test and falls to one side*

Meningeal Signs

- *Meningeal signs: + stiff neck, + Kernig, + Brudzinski*

Straight Leg Raising

- *Straight leg raise: + R, neg on L is how to chart the straight leg raise test*

Extremities

Depending on the case, you may need to comment on joints in general (lupus or rheumatoid arthritis) or on specific joints (an acute injury). Some examples:

- R wrist-swollen, erythematous, decreased active or passive ROM
- Joints-no swelling/ erythema / tenderness/ full ROM
- L elbow-no swelling/ red/ tender/ limited ROM
- MCP's and PIP's-red, swollen and tender bilaterally
- If a patient presents with right knee problems, for example, while considering a differential diagnosis for knee pain, take into consideration as well hip problems that can refer to the knee and present as knee pain.
- A sample Patient Note for normal lumbosacral and lower extremities is presented below:
- Lower back: no obvious deformities or signs of trauma; no spinous process or paraspinal tenderness and full ROM to flexion, extension and lateral rotation.
- Lower extremities: ROM WNL, motor 5/5 , B/L, DTR 2+ (patellar, Achilles) sensation intact to sharp and dull B/L
- Gait: WNL
- Peripheral Pulses: 2+ DP, PT

PSYCHIATRIC EXAMINATION

Below is the documentation of the normal version of the psychiatric examination:

- **GA:** Patient appears well-groomed, alert, and oriented to person, place, and time (A&O x 3), Speech fluid and goal-directed; Recent and remote memory intact; Attention and concentration unimpaired; Mood euthymic; affect c/w mood; No abnormal perceptions: hallucinations, delusions, or paranoia; No suicidal/homicidal ideation or intent; Judgment/insight are intact.

DIFFERENTIAL DIAGNOSIS

An important component of the Patient Note is the differential diagnosis filled in with all supporting data. There are 3 available spaces for differential diagnosis.

- List diagnoses in order from **most likely** to **least likely**, typing only one diagnosis per line.
- Your diagnoses should be written **based on the hypotheses generated from the introductory information**, and then further refined during the history-taking and physical examination.
- Your diagnoses must be supported by entering the positives and negative findings from the history and physical examination.
  - Include the relevant supporting factors in the appropriate spaces of your Patient Note (up to 8 rows for each diagnosis).
  - Attempt to document 8 total findings for the first diagnosis, and 4 for each additional diagnosis chosen. Since time is limited, you are not expected to fill in 8 rows of history findings and 8 rows of physical findings for every differential diagnosis.

Helpful Tips for Differential Diagnosis

- Write the most likely diagnosis first.
- Use only those abbreviations listed on the usmle.org website. If you are unsure about the abbreviation, type out the full name.
- Write diseases, not symptoms (congestive heart failure, not shortness of breath).
- Include only diagnoses that can be supported by the patient's symptoms, past medical history and/or physical exam findings.
- You may list fewer than 3 diagnoses in certain cases. Make sure that every diagnosis listed can be supported with history and physical findings.
- "Noncompliance with medicine" and "medication side effect" can be legitimate diagnoses.

DIAGNOSTIC WORKUP

The last component of the Patient Note includes immediate plans for a diagnostic workup. Here, you will carefully correlate the list of all immediate diagnostic tests that you will perform to further confirm your differential diagnosis. Guidelines for writing the workup include the following:

- You are given up to 8 rows on this section; if more then 8 tests are appropriate for a given case, group similar tests as 1 row such as: blood & urine tests, radiologic tests.
- Include prohibited physical exam maneuvers that are relevant to the case.
- Do not mention treatments, counseling, hospitalizations, referrals, or consultations
- Use acceptable abbreviations
- For a case with no workup, write "*No studies indicated*"; do not leave it blank.
- Do not list test panels or groups, e.g., LFTS but instead list AST, ALT
- You will not receive credit for listing allowed physical exam maneuvers you would have done if the encounter had been longer

PATIENT NOTE TIME MANAGEMENT

If you leave the patient encounter early, you may use the additional time for typing the note. On rare occasions the computer may malfunction. If that happens, you will be asked to hand-write the Patient Note by using the same format. Go to usmle.org and familiarize yourself with the Patient Note format and **practice, practice, practice!** Here are a few tips to help improve your practice performance:

- Use either the mouse or tab to move to the next box
- To highlight a single word, drag or double click the left mouse button. To highlight an entire line drag using the left mouse button (select all will select the whole section, not just the wanted line).
- To copy/paste, highlight and then use the right mouse button or CTRL C and CTRL V
- Leave out commas when it does not interfere with understanding
- When justifying the differential diagnosis, enter relevant information under the first differential and then copy and paste what is relevant into the other diagnosis.

Remember that **time is of the essence**; listing **phrase format** (examples given through this chapter) is preferred over narrative paragraph to save time. To earn more points, we suggest that you type the following first:

- Chief complaint and HPI
- Relevant PMH
- Differential diagnosis with justification
- Diagnostic studies
- Physical examination

Depending on the time you have left, add additional information collected during the encounter from the PMH.

PRACTICE CASE

Now that you have completed the chapter on the Patient Note, you should be able to write an excellent note. First, go back to the **original practice case in chapter 2**, and review the history and physical examination. Then go to **usmle.org** and type your Note for the case. Remember to set a timer for the 10 minutes allotted.

Once you have completed your Note, compare it to the one below. Given the time constraints of the exam, your Note will be somewhat shorter.

PATIENT NOTE FOR PRACTICE CASE: SEVERE ABDOMINAL PAIN

Patient Note

History

CC: 35 yo F c/o severe abdominal pain

HPI: RLQ, x6hrs, 10/10, sharp, stabbing, sudden, constant, progressive, no radiation, no precipitating factors. Aggrav by movement and deep breaths. No relief with Advil. + vaginal spotting and nausea. No vomiting, diarrhea, anorexia, fever, vag discharge, or urinary changes.

PMH: no h/o CC or trauma. h/o UTI, PID. Hosp/surg for appendectomy

ObGyn: G0P0, LMP 6 wks ago

Meds: Advil prn, No Rx. NKDA.

FHx: No h/o CC or illnesses

SH: Sexually active with bf, 20 M partners x 10 years, occ condoms, HIV not tested. No tobacco or rec drugs. Occ EtOH

Physical Examination

VS: 98.6 F, RR: 19/min, HR 100/min, BP 120/78 mm Hg

General: Pt lying in fetal position in acute distress

Abd: RLQ scar. +BSx4Q, tympanic x4Q, soft, not distended. + RLQ tenderness, + rebound. No CVA tenderness. No hepato-splenomegaly

Data Interpretation

DIAGNOSIS 1. ECTOPIC PREGNANCY

History Support	Physical Exam Support
Acute RLQ pain	Afebrile
LMP 6 wks ago	RLQ tenderness
Vag spotting	Rebound
Nausea	No CVA tenderness
h/o PID	
Age 35	
h/o ruptured appendix	
No vag D/C	

DIAGNOSIS 2. OVARIAN TORSION/RUPTURED OVARIAN CYST

History Support	Physical Exam Support
Acute RLQ pain	Afebrile
h/o ruptured appendix	RLQ tenderness
Progressive sharp pain	Rebound
Nausea	No CVA tenderness
LMP 6 wks ago	
Vaginal spotting	
No vag D/C	

DIAGNOSIS 3. PID

History Support	Physical Exam Support
h/o PID	RLQ tenderness
Multiple sex partners	No CVA tenderness
Inconsistent condom use	
Abdominal pain	
Vag spotting	
Nausea	

Diagnostic Studies

Pelvic/rectal exam

B-HCG, CBC w diff, ESR, CRP

Pelvic U/S with color flow Doppler

Cervical swab: GC, chlamydia, C/S

Differential Diagnosis   7

Each standardized patient (SP) encounter requires test takers to exhibit capable data-gathering through the history and focused physical examination. The task is to generate hypotheses, leading to the establishment of a differential diagnosis.

Generating hypotheses begins outside the exam room with the posted patient information: patient's age, chief complaint or reason for the visit, location of the encounter, and vital signs, e.g., *a 58-year-old man presents to the clinic with chest pain of several hours' duration.*

This "doorway information" sets the stage for the encounter by enabling you to think of possible common diagnoses before the start of the encounter. Possible common reasons for chest pain in a 58-year-old include:

- Acute coronary syndrome, MI
- Acute coronary syndrome, unstable angina
- Pneumonia
- GERD
- Costochondritis

If this patient presented with fever, the initial list of hypotheses might be:

- Pneumonia
- Pleuritis
- MI
- Costochondritis

Once inside the exam room, pursue a line of questioning mindful of the diagnoses you are considering. Continue generating hypotheses while you add or remove possible diagnoses. Return to the chief complaint and chronology. Careful consideration of hypotheses will lead to a productive and sharply focused physical exam.

During the examination, continue asking questions about the history of present illness (HPI) as you identify abnormalities. The list of hypotheses will have changed from the time you read the doorway information to the point of presenting your ideas with diagnostic and therapeutic plans.

Suppose a 20-year-old man complains of sudden onset shortness of breath and his vitals prior to your entering the room reveal respiratory rate 40/min and pulse 118/min. In that situation, you may generate a differential diagnosis such as:

- Pneumothorax
- Acute allergic reaction
- Asthma attack
- Pulmonary embolus
- Pneumonia

If this patient denies fever and cough, pneumonia is very unlikely; it will remain at the bottom of your list. If he has a peanut allergy and just ate Thai food for lunch, he may be having an acute allergic reaction. As you complete your history, you'll want to ask about allergies, history of asthma, trauma, and family history.

If this patient is a healthy young man who arrived home yesterday from a European backpacking trip with his friends, pulmonary embolus would be at the top of your differential diagnosis list. The history he would give you might be that he woke up this morning, got out of bed, and suddenly became short of breath. He might also say that he slept the entire flight home because he was so exhausted from hiking every day.

As you can see from the case of this 20-year-old with dyspnea, **pertinent positives** will help support the likely diagnosis for your case. **Pertinent negatives** will either help eliminate a differential totally or make it much less likely to be the primary diagnosis for the case. Asking the right questions and finding the right positives and negatives will help in diagnosis selection and will be used in the patient note as the findings to justify the differentials chosen.

Another example will help solidify this concept:

> A 30-year-old woman complains of fatigue. She admits to recent weight gain and sleeping more hours than she normally did during the past several years. She denies problems adjusting to temperature changes, and any changes in her skin and hair texture.

These facts make it more likely that the diagnosis for the case is major depressive disorder and less likely that it is a case of hypothyroidism. Nevertheless, hypothyroidism should still be used as a differential for this case.

You are also told that she eats a healthy diet that includes red meat and denies heavy menses. Since there is no evidence of anemia, it should not be considered at all for this case.

Finally, stop and review one last time the approach to differential diagnosis. Now return to your patient note for the chapter 2 practice case and be sure that you can identify and understand the relevant positives from history and physical examination. Next, be sure you understand the included examples of pertinent negatives. Recognize that although the patient has a history of PID and current risk factors, it is listed as the third differential since the patient does not have a vaginal discharge or fever. The case facts you use to determine your diagnoses will be the justifications used in your patient note. The more organized your thought process and approach, the easier it will be to write an excellent patient note. Also remember that the selected differentials are not the only possible ones to use for this case. Others to consider would be threatened/incomplete abortion, urinary tract infection, or even endometriosis.

COMMON ERRORS IN THE DIFFERENTIAL DIAGNOSIS PROCESS

Determining the proper differential diagnosis is one of the keys to passing the Step 2 CS exam. Four common errors may occur.

Error 1. Skipping steps in data-gathering

When generating hypotheses, the history is the most important source of information. Fixating on narrow or incomplete data from initial answers can lead to an erroneous line of questioning with failure to elicit more relevant symptoms.

Solution

- Keep the focus on the generated hypotheses.
- Ask questions leading to or eliminating diagnoses. If you ask, "What other symptoms have you had?," the SP will respond with, "What do you want to know, doctor?"
- Ask about other concerns.
- Always ask for clarification of the events in the HPI.
- Listen carefully to a patient's complete answer before moving on.

Error 2. Using wrong information

Even when you have asked the right question and believe you have eliminated possible diagnoses for the right reasons, it is still possible to use wrong information in your conclusions. For example, in response to the question, "Do you smoke?" the patient says, "No." But had you asked, "Do you use tobacco?" the patient's answer might have been, "I don't smoke, but I do chew."

Solution

- Clarify answers to ensure your correct understanding. ("You said that you have never smoked. Have you used any other tobacco product, like snuff or chew?")
- Consider an answer's completeness and accuracy in the context of the patient's age, gender, or other history. ("You said that both your parents, your siblings, and your wife all smoke, but that you don't. Have you ever used any other tobacco product, like snuff or chew?")

Error 3. Restricting or limiting the problem

It is incorrect to limit or restrict a differential diagnosis based upon preconceived assumptions.

You may prematurely bring closure to a sequence of valid questions. For example, a patient whom you believe is using illegal drugs because of general appearance may lead you away from asking key questions and failing to believe there is no history of illegal drug use.

Solution

- Perform the evaluation based on presented information without making wrong assumptions.
- Be objective in your assessment of the patient's clinical status. Don't let physical appearances influence your establishment of rapport.

Error 4. Giving up on a problem too soon

One of the challenges on the Step CS exam is to have a patient who speaks very little, is angry, or has difficulty communicating information. What behaviors are useful in these situations to enable you to obtain all necessary information?

Solution

- Facilitate communication by encouraging the patient. Repeat or paraphrase what is said to enhance your understanding of the problem. Summaries are extremely helpful, even short ones.

- Use more closed-ended questions; yes/no answers provide information when patients are unable to provide longer answers.
- Most important, demonstrate even more caring and concern about the patient's health with verbal and nonverbal reassurances.
- Start the physical examination earlier than usual. Clues will be present as you examine the patient and continue to ask questions as you move from one region to the next.

Another challenge is generating differentials diagnoses for psychiatric complaints. Two common examples are depression and anxiety.

A differential diagnosis for depression:
- MDD (major depressive disorder)
- GAD (general anxiety disorder) (depression and anxiety are closely related – if you consider one, list the other)
- Hypothyroidism
- Somatization disorder

A diagnostic plan for depression includes screening tests for common chronic diseases: anemia, renal failure, diabetes mellitus, hypothyroidism, chronic liver disease, or a chronic infection. It is of key importance, and a patient's confidence will increase, if you carefully consider the patient's presenting somatic symptoms. One simple test to assess them; for instance, an abdominal U/S to evaluate abdominal pain can be of therapeutic benefit.

A differential diagnosis for anxiety:
- GAD
- MDD
- Hyperthyroidism
- Somatization disorder

A diagnostic plan for GAD is similar to the one for MDD, i.e., screening tests for common chronic diseases: anemia, renal failure, diabetes mellitus, hyperthyroidism, chronic liver disease, or a chronic infection.

Generating an accurate differential diagnosis is a key component of the Step 2 CS exam and an important skill in being a safe and competent physician.

GATHERING DATA TO SUPPORT THE DIAGNOSIS

The following section provides a few common cases, along with the relevant history, physical findings, and appropriate tests that would support a particular diagnosis.

This is intended only as a guide to help you learn how to support your diagnosis and select an appropriate and relevant work up. It is not an exhaustive list.

CC	Diagnosis	HPI	PMH	PE Findings	WorkUp
HEENT					
40 yo man c/o of dizziness and hearing loss	Meniere disease	Episodic spells of vertigo that lasts 4–5 hrs Fluctuating unilateral hearing loss Aura & ear fullness Nausea & vomiting Tinnitus	Hyperlipidemia/DM/MI FHx hearing problems	Low frequency sensorineural hearing loss; with nl hearing between attacks. Rinne test (b/l) consistent with sensorineural deficit on affected ear; Weber (b/l) lateralization to contralateral affected ear. Gait problems	Audiometry Vestibular testing Electrocochleography (ECochG) for endolymphatic hydrops VDRL/RPR/FTA-ab Brain MRI Dix-Hallpike maneuver
40 yo man c/o of dizziness and hearing loss	Otitis media	Ear pain (otalgia) Pain behind the ear Suppuration of retained secretions (otorrhea) Decreased hearing typically unilateral	Preceding URI h/o seasonal allergic rhinitis Recurrent otitis media	Conductive hearing loss Rinne test (b/l) on affected ear, consistent with conductive hearing loss on affected ear Weber test (b/l): lateralization to affected ear Erythematous or opacified TM Bulging or perforated TM Fever or facial palsy	CBC w/diff Otomicroscopy Fiberoptic nasopharyngoscopy
40 yo man c/o of dizziness nausea and vomiting	Vestibular neuronitis	Vertigo Nausea aggravated by head movements Lasts for days Vomiting Gait problems	h/o hearing impairment h/o vertigo h/o URI	Gait instability Hearing impairment Weber and Rinne (b/l)	MRI/MRA
35 yo man c/o dizziness	Labyrinthitis	Vertigo Ringing in ears (tinnitus) Nausea/vomiting	Recent URI	Examine ear with otoscope Check for nystagmus	Audiometry

CC	Diagnosis	HPI	PMH	PE Findings	WorkUp
Middle-aged man c/o pink eye	Conjunctivitis	Redness and swelling of the conjunctiva Sensation of foreign body in the eye Skin itching and watery discharge from both eyes NL VA and no photophobia	h/o seasonal or specific allergies h/o URI h/o STDs (gonorrhea, chlamydia) h/o Sjogren Sdr. h/o wearing contact lenses h/o swimming	Purulent discharge from one or both eyes Watery discharge from one or both eyes Diffuse redness of conjunctiva Normal vision and no other eye findings Normal fundoscopic exam	Rapid test for Adenoviral Conjunctivitis PCR and culture of swabbed specimens
25 yo man c/o facial pain	Sinusitis	Thick, green nasal discharge Cough that is worse at night Dull, constant headache Pain worse when tilting head forward	h/o asthma	Fever Tenderness on palpation of sinuses	-
67 yo man c/o difficulty swallowing	Esophagitis (medication induced)	Retro-sternal pain or heartburn h/o difficulty swallowing (dysphagia); painful swallowing (odynophagia); vomiting blood (hematemesis) Abd pain Weight loss Increased age	h/o GERD h/o H. pylori Obesity Pregnancy or exogenous estrogen h/o NSAIDs, AB, bisphosphonates, etc.	-	UGI endoscopy Ba esophagram
67 yo man with difficulty swallowing	Esophageal cancer	Dysphagia: solids > liquids Sensation of food stuck in throat Weight loss	h/o smoking and alcoholism h/o GERD Obesity	LAD	Ba esophagram UGI endoscopy and biopsy CT of chest and upper abd PET scan for metastasis CXR
57 yo woman c/o difficulty swallowing	Plummer-Vinson syndrome	Soreness or inflammation of the tongue (Glossitis) Inflammation of the corners of the mouth (Angular Cheilitis) Painful swallowing (Odynophagia)	h/o iron deficiency anemia Post-menopausal Vegan diet	Cheilosis Pallor	CBC Upper endoscopy
18 yo woman c/o sore throat	Pharyngitis	Runny nose Cough Headache Hoarse voice	Recent viral infection	Fever	Throat swab

CC	Diagnosis	HPI	PMH	PE Findings	WorkUp
17 yo girl c/o sore throat	Infectious mononucleosis	Sore throat Fatigue Pain aggravated by swallowing (Odynophagia)	h/o enlarged lymph nodes (Lymphade-nopathy) Sick contacts	Fever Pharyngitis (exudative or not) Hepatosplenomegaly Lymphadenopathy	CBC w/diff ESR Monospot test
35 yo woman c/o palpitations	Hyperthyroidism	Heat intolerance Unintentional weight loss Irritability Brittle hair Diarrhea	FHx of thyroid disease	Hand tremors Tachycardia Hyperventilation Increased DTR	TSH, T3, T4 Thyroid uptake scan
Pulmonary					
Middle-aged man c/o severe chest pain and SOB	Pulmonary embolism	Sudden onset of SOB (Dyspnea) SOB when lying flat (Orthopnea) Dyspnea at rest or at exertion (73%) Cough Blood-tinged sputum (Hemoptysis) Sudden onset of pleuritic pain Calf or thigh pain and/or swelling	h/o smoking h/o immobilization or recent long flight Profession that involves prolonged sitting (e.g. cab or truck driver)	Hypertension/hypotension Tachypnea Tachycardia Wheezing Calf or thigh swelling	CXR EKG ABG Spiral CT VQ scan D-dimer (only when low probability)
Middle-aged man c/o acute shortness of breath and agitation	COPD Exacerbation	Acute exacerbation of SOB Chronic h/o SOB Chronic h/o of productive cough	h/o lung disease h/o smoking	Tachypnea Decreased chest excursion Barrel chest Hyperresonance (b/l)	PFTs CXR Pulse oximetry ABG
Middle-aged man c/o acute shortness of breath and agitation	Spontaneous Pneumothorax	Sudden onset SOB Pleuritic chest pain Tall and thin male	Previous episodes of spontaneous pneumothorax	Tachypnea Decreased chest excursion on affected side Diminished breath sounds Hyperresonance	AP and lateral CXR
67 yo woman c/o significant SOB	Cor Pulmonale	Chronic h/o SOB SOB on exertion Exertional syncope Exertional angina B/l swelling of LE in past several wks	Long-standing h/o lung disease h/o smoking	S3/S4 Split S2	CXR ECG Echo Pulse oximetry ABG PFTs

CC	Diagnosis	HPI	PMH	PE Findings	WorkUp
Elderly man c/o worsening dyspnea on exertion	COPD	Chronic h/o SOB Chronic h/o of productive cough Morning white sputum	Long-standing h/o smoking Chronic h/o lung disease	Tachypnea Prolonged expirations Distant breath sounds Barrel chest	PFTs CXR Pulse oximetry ABG
Elderly man c/o worsening dyspnea on exertion and productive cough	TB	Chronic h/o SOB Chronic h/o of productive purulent cough h/o blood in sputum (Hemoptysis) Night sweats Weight loss Fatigue	Foreign born/travel h/o smoking HIV Immunosuppressed status Exposure to TB (Health worker)	Fever Tachypnea Cachexia	PFTs CXR Pulse oximetry ABG TB sputum Gram stain and culture TB blood test CBC w dif Blood culture
Elderly man c/o worsening dyspnea on exertion and productive cough	Chronic asthma	h/o SOB early in life Aggravated at night/early morning	H/x of allergies H/x of smoking Exposure to second-hand smoke	Tachypnea Prolonged expirations Diffuse wheezing Increased vocal fremitus Intercostal retractions	PFTs CXR ABG
Elderly man c/o worsening dyspnea on exertion and productive cough	Bronchogenic carcinoma (central airway obstruction)	Cough with purulent sputum Slowly progressive SOB (Dyspnea) Purulent sputum Unintended weight loss Hemoptysis	h/o smoking	Tachypnea Prolonged expirations Wheezing	CXR Chest CT Bronchoscopy
65 yo man c/o cough	Lung cancer	Hemoptysis Dyspnea Unintended weight loss Fatigue Productive cough	h/o smoking FHx of cancer	Wheezing on lung exam	CXR Sputum Gram stain and culture Chest CT
60 yo man c/o chest pain and cough	Pneumonia	Cough SOB Purulent sputum Chest pain	Recent viral prodrome	Febrile Mild respiratory distress Tachypnea Crackles Areas of lung consolidation	CXR Blood culture Sputum Gram stain & culture CBC w/diff

CC	Diagnosis	HPI	PMH	PE Findings	WorkUp
60 yo man c/o chest pain and cough	**Pleural effusion**	Pleuritic chest pain (aggravated by deep breaths or motion) Cough SOB	Recent viral prodrome	Febrile Mild respiratory distress Dullness Egophony	CXR Chest U/S Pleural fluid cell count/cytology Histology/culture LDH/pH Sputum culture
Cardiovascular					
53 yo man c/o recurrent chest pain, dyspnea, and anxiety	**MI**	Diaphoresis Crushing retrosternal pain >20 min Location: chest, neck, lower jaw, and down left arm FHx heart disease SOB	Smoker h/o angina or MI	Pale and diaphoretic Tachycardia Hemodynamic instability	EKG CK-MB Cardiac troponin Echo
53 yo man c/o recurrent chest pain, dyspnea, and anxiety	**Angina pectoris/stable angina**	Pain <20 min Gradual onset Quality: discomfort rather than pain/pressure/ heaviness/tightness/ constriction Location: center or left of chest Aggravated by exertion Alleviated by rest No change with respiration or position SOB	h/o high cholesterol h/o HTN	Levine sign High BP S3 or S4	EKG Stress test
Middle-aged man c/o severe chest pain	**Aortic dissection**	"Tearing" chest pain Back pain Acute onset	h/o high BP/HTN h/o Cocaine use Congenital factors like Marfan, Turner, or Noonan syndromes	Hypertension BP asymmetry on UE UE pulselessness Hemodynamic instability	CXR Transesophageal echo CT scan Urine toxicology
Middle-aged man c/o severe chest pain	**Cocaine-induced ACS**	Chest pain Agitation	Cocaine Myocarditis Vasculitis	Hypertension Arrhythmias Nasal septum perforation	EKG/CK-MB Troponins I/T Urine toxicology

CC	Diagnosis	HPI	PMH	PE Findings	WorkUp
67 yo woman c/o significant dyspnea	CHF/ pulmonary edema	SOB PND Orthopnea Cough (pink frothy sputum) Noncompliant with medication Swelling of the legs x past several wks	h/o HTN MI	JVD Peripheral edema Rales at the base of the lung S3 gallop	ECG Echo BNP Troponins CXR
67 yo woman c/o significant dyspnea	Myocarditis	Chest pain Fatigue Swelling of the legs x past several wks	h/o URI	Tachycardia Gallop Peripheral edema	CBC with diff ESR/CRP ECG CXR Echo
67 yo woman c/o significant dyspnea	Atrial fibrillation	Palpitations Irregularly/irregular pulse Lightheadedness Anxiety	h/o cardiomyopathy h/o HTN	Pallor Diaphoresis Irregular heart rate Dyspneic	ECG Holter 24–48 hr Event recorder
60 yo man c/o chest pain and cough	Pericarditis	Sharp pleuritic chest pain alleviated by leaning forward (sitting) Persistent fever	Recent viral prodrome	Febrile Mild respiratory distress Pericardial friction rub Rash on skin	ECG Echo CXR Blood cultures
Middle-aged man c/o palpitation and chest pain	Mitral valve prolapse (MVP)	Chest pain Palpitation Dyspnea Chest pressure Exercise intolerance Dizziness Anxiety disorder	h/o HTN h/o arrhythmia Pulmonary edema	Hypertension Arrhythmias CV systolic murmurs and non-ejection clicks Narrow A-P chest diameter Scoliosis and loss of kyphosis of spine	EKG/CK-MB Troponin I/T Transthoracic echo Doppler echo CMR (CV magnetic resonance)
Middle-aged man c/o dizziness	Drug induced orthostatic hypotension	Dizziness Syncope Sx onset after standing or eating	h/o angina h/o stroke h/o supine HTN h/o HTN medication	Pallor Diaphoresis Hypotension Tachycardia	Monitor orthostatic/ supine/and sitting BP
69 yo man c/o lightheadedness	Orthostatic hypotension from dehydration	Fatigue Palpitations Profuse sweating Nausea	Diarrhea Excessive exercise Decreased fluid intake	Orthostatic hypotension Pale	BUN and Creatinine CBC Electrolytes

CC	Diagnosis	HPI	PMH	PE Findings	WorkUp
Endocrinology					
Patient c/o palpitation, and anxiety	Insulinoma	Severe episodes of fasting or postprandial hypoglycemia Palpitations, diaphoresis, and tremulousness Weight gain Confusion Visual changes Unusual behavior	FHx MEN1	Peripheral tremor	Blood glucose Plasma insulin and GLP-1 level Abd CT/MRI/U/S
Patient c/o palpitations, and anxiety	Hypoglycemia	Symptoms consistent with hypoglycemia (tremor, palpitations, anxiety, sweating, hunger, paresthesia) Low blood glucose level Symptoms remit after glucose is raised	Repetitive similar episodes during fasting Insulin or other DM tx h/o alcohol use Hormone deficiency (cortisol glucagon epinephrine) h/o insulinoma	Peripheral tremor	Blood glucose level Insulin level C-peptide level BHOB level Proinsulin level Sulfonylurea and meglitinide screen
ObGyn and Urology					
38 yo woman c/o vaginal discharge	**Bacterial vaginosis**	Grayish white thin watery discharge Malodorous Post-menstrual onset	IUD Douching practice Recent antibiotics Menopause Multiple sexual partners Unprotected sex	-	Pelvic exam Wet /saline prep Vaginal pH Whiff test
38 yo woman c/o vaginal discharge	**Trichomonal vaginitis**	Copious green/yellow frothy discharge Malodorous Pruritic Dyspareunia Dysuria Post-coital bleeding	Unprotected intercourse Multiple sexual partners IUD/smoker	-	Pelvic exam Wet/saline prep Vaginal pH
38 yo woman c/o vaginal discharge	Candida vaginitis	White, thick, cheesy discharge Odorless Pruritic Dyspareunia Dysuria	Previous episodes Recent antibiotics Diabetes/pregnancy HIV/OCP	-	Pelvic exam KOH prep Vaginal pH

CC	Diagnosis	HPI	PMH	PE Findings	WorkUp
48 yo woman c/o vaginal discharge	**Atrophic vaginitis**	Vaginal dryness Dysuria/urgency/frequency Hot flashes Post-coital bleeding	Sleep disturbances Osteoporosis Pelvic organ prolapse Tamoxifen/lupron Menopause	-	Pelvic exam FSH Estradiol Vaginal smear
38 yo woman c/o heavy vaginal bleeding	**Abnormal uterine bleeding (AUB)**	Abn bleeding >6 mos (frequency/regularity/duration/volume) Brown-stain bleeding color Dysmenorrhea Reproductive age Not pregnant Fatigue	Abn bleeding >6 mos h/o thyroid disease Not taking local or systemic gonadosteroids Not taking any other medication OCP (estrogen/progesterone) Systemic disorders of hemostasis Ovulatory disorders Primary disorders of endometrium	Tachycardia Pallor	Pelvic exam CBC Extraction of HB (alkaline hematin method) Pictorial blood loss assessment charts
38 yo woman c/o heavy vaginal bleeding	**Endometriosis**	Abn bleeding Pelvic pain h/o infertility Urinary urgency/frequency Dyspareunia Dysmenorrhea Dyschezia	FHx endometriosis FHx infertility	-	Pelvic exam Abd U/S Transvaginal U/S Abd CT
38 yo woman c/o heavy vaginal bleeding	**Spontaneous abortion**	Confirmed pregnancy Sudden onset of vaginal bleeding Abd pain and contractions NSAID use	Advanced maternal age h/o smoking Cocaine use Previous spontaneous abortions Prolonged time to achieve pregnancy Maternal infection	Fever	Pelvic exam Abd U/S Beta HCG Folate level RhD level CBC w diff

CC	Diagnosis	HPI	PMH	PE Findings	WorkUp
45 yo woman c/o abnormal vaginal bleeding	**Cervical cancer**	Pelvic pain Dyspareunia Bleeding after sexual intercourse Weight loss Anorexia	h/o HPV infection Smoker Multiple sexual partners Inconsistent condom use OCP use over 10 years	-	Pelvic exam Pap smear
18 yo woman c/o irregular menses	**Stress-induced amenorrhea**	No menses for 3 mos Started college 3 mos ago	Mother also experienced amenorrhea during stressful times	-	bHCG Testosterone and estrogen levels Abd U/S
30 yo woman c/o amenorrhea	**Prolactinoma**	Galactorrhea Oligomenorrhea/ amenorrhea Loss of axillary and pubic hair Headache	-	Loss of peripheral vision	Prolactin level Brain MRI
48 yo woman c/o amenorrhea for few mos	**Menopause**	Amenorrhea for 12 mos Hot flashes Vaginal dryness Sleep disturbances Mood imbalance New onset of depression Decline in cognitive function Dyspareunia Joint pain Breast pain, tenderness	Irregular menstrual cycles >4 yrs before final menstrual period Progressive gradual decrease in menstrual bleeding or very heavy and prolonged bleeding FHx early menopause h/o smoking could affect an earlier onset of menopause h/o hysterectomy with ovarian conservation h/o menstrual migraine	Increased age and wrinkling of the skin	Pelvic exam Inhibin B FSH and LH Estradiol level AMH level(anti-mullerian hormone) AFC (ovarian antral follicular count) Transvaginal and pelvic U/S TSH

CC	Diagnosis	HPI	PMH	PE Findings	WorkUp
Middle-aged woman c/o amenorrhea for few wks	**Pregnancy**	Amenorrhea Nausea w/or w/o vomiting Breast enlargement and tenderness Increased frequency in urination w/o dysuria Fatigue Mild uterine cramping/ discomfort w/o bleeding Constipation and heart burn Nasal congestion Sexually active Reproductive age Physiologic pruritus (scalp, vulva, anus, abd, skin) Increased or decreased hair growth Hirsutism Androgenic alopecia Constipation and bloating, increased flatus, hemorrhoids and incontinence Increased salivation Food cravings and aversion Mood changes	New onset of GERD or aggravation Hx. of previous pregnancy	Changes in skin: increased pigmentations (face, linea alba areola), nevi, melasma, striae gravidarum Vascular changes: spider angiomata, palmar erythema, varicosities, vascular tumors, hemorrhoids Enlarged uterus on abd palpation Gingivitis	Urine and Blood BHCG Serum ALT/AST/ bilirubin Abd, pelvic, and transvaginal U/S Pelvic exam Asses fetal heart activity with Doppler devices CBC
26 yo woman c/o difficulty getting pregnant	**Polycystic ovary syndrome**	Dysmenorrhea Unintentional weight gain Hirsutism	Pelvic pain DM II h/o OSA Hx ovarian cysts Similar symptoms in aunt G0P0 h/o excessive acne	Facial acne Patches of thin, darker velvety skin Obese abdomen Hirsutism	Pelvic exam Serum HCG Pelvic US Androgen levels Serum insulin level Homocysteine level
30 yo woman c/o dysuria	**Urethritis**	Urinary urgency Urinary frequency Difficulty starting urination Itching, pain, burning and discomfort in urination and genitalia Dysmenorrhea Vaginal d/c	Active with multiple sexual partners Inconsistent condom use h/o PID	-	Pelvic exam U/A

CC	Diagnosis	HPI	PMH	PE Findings	WorkUp
55 yo woman c/o urinary incontinence	**Urge incontinence**	Sudden uncontrolled urine loss associated with a strong desire to void	h/o UTI h/o DM h/o BPH (men) Surgeries: C section (women), prostate (men) Pregnancy/delivery	No abd. tenderness No CVA tenderness	Genital and pelvic exams UA Cystometry Post void residual volume Pelvic or abd U/S
55 yo woman c/o urinary incontinence	**Stress incontinence**	Involuntary urine loss while coughing, laughing, lifting, sneezing	h/o constipation h/o urinary incontinence Multiple pregnancies/deliveries h/o smoking h/o prostatectomy (in men)	No abd. tenderness No CVA tenderness	Genital and pelvic exams UA Cystometry Post-void residual volume Pelvic or abd U/S
70 yo man c/o nocturia	**Benign prostatic hyperplasia**	Urinary urgency Urinary hesitancy Urinary frequency Urinary incontinence Weak urine stream Straining to void Sense of incomplete emptying Terminal dribbling	FH	Abd exam WNL	Prostate exam PSA Transrectal U/S
70 yo man c/o hematuria	**Prostate cancer**	Back pain Fatigue Weight loss Increased urinary frequency and urgency Difficulty starting and maintaining stream of urine Nocturia Dysuria	Diet high in processed meat Father with h/o prostate cancer	Obese Abd exam WNL	Prostate exam PSA Transrectal U/S
60 yo man c/o hematuria	**Bladder cancer**	Dysuria Increased urinary frequency Urinary urgency	Heavy long-time smoker Occupation: hair dresser	No findings on abd exam	UA Urine cytology cystoscopy

CC	Diagnosis	HPI	PMH	PE Findings	WorkUp
60 yo man c/o hematuria	Renal cell carcinoma	Flank pain Unintentional weight loss Fatigue	Smoker Fhx of kidney cancer Excess acetaminophen use Occupational exposure to asbestos HTN	Obesity noted Abd mass noted	U/A Abd CT
37 yo man c/o groin pain	Testicular torsion	Young adolescent men Sudden onset of severe testicular pain Unilateral Pain radiates to lower back Nausea and vomiting	Onset during physical exertion	-	Genital exam Doppler U/S of scrotum
37 yo Man/ Woman c/o increasing flank pain	Nephrolithiasis	Sudden onset excruciating back&flank pain Colicky pain (restlessness) Radiation to groin or abdomen Nausea/vomiting Anorexia Dysuria	h/o kidney stone h/o dehydration High protein & sodium diet Overweight	Fever CVA tenderness	Helical renal CT U/A for Ca, oxalates, uric acid Renal US
37 yo Man/ Woman c/o flank pain and fever	Pyelonephritis	Dysuria Fever Nausea and vomiting Urinary frequency (Polyuria) Urinary urgency Hematuria Chills	h/o recurrent UTI h/o BPH (men)	Fever CVA tenderness	U/A Urine culture Renal U/S
Abdomen					
45 yo woman c/o right-sided abdominal pain	Acute cholecystitis (biliary colic)	Acute, persistent RUQ pain Pain related to fatty foods Radiation to R scapula Associated with N/V Fever	OCP use Obese DM FHx of gallbladder disease Multiparity	Patient appears uncomfortable Overweight Fever Tenderness in RUQ Murphy's sign Tachycardic	CBC w/diff Abd U/S AST, ALT, ALP, bilirubin ERCP HIDA

CC	Diagnosis	HPI	PMH	PE Findings	WorkUp
41 yo woman c/o acute painful abdominal distress	Pancreatitis	Severe and persistent epigastric pain Radiates to the back Alleviated by sitting up or bending forward Nausea/vomiting	h/o binge alcohol consumption h/o gallstones	Pt appears ill and very uncomfortable Epigastric tenderness Rebound guarding Cullen/Grey Turner sign Febrile Tachycardic	Serum amylase/ lipase Trypsinogen activation peptide CRP/ALT/AST Abd x-ray Abd U/S Abd CT
53 yo man c/o recurrent chest pain, dyspnea, and anxiety	GERD	Postprandial discomfort Aggravated when supine Heartburn Regurgitations Dysphagia Chest pain Nausea	Obesity h/o smoking	Wheezing	Esophageal PH monitoring EGD
41 yo woman c/o acute painful abdominal distress	Peptic ulcer disease	Epigastric pain and fullness Pain is persistent Nausea/Vomiting Hematemesis Melena	h/o NSAIDs use h/o previous *H. pylori*	Pt appears uncomfortable Epigastric tenderness	Endoscopy Fecal occult blood
46 yo woman c/o abdominal pain and nausea	Gastritis	Epigastric pain Aggravated by food intake Alleviated by Tums Nausea and vomiting	h/o *H. pylori* h/o infections and autoimmune disease	Tenderness in epigastric area	UGI endoscopy *H. pylori* testing Serum pepsinogen (PG I and II) Antibodies to intrinsic factor, parietal cells, and *H. pylori*
68 yo woman c/o chills, nausea, and abdominal pain;	Gastroenteritis (Norovirus)	Nonbloody diarrhea Vomiting/nausea Crampy abd pain Onset in winter season Malaise	Sick contacts	Pt appears frail and uncomfortable Fever Diffuse abd. tenderness Dehydration	Blood culture FOB Fecal leukocyte Fecal lactoferrin
68 yo woman c/o chills, nausea, and abdominal pain	Hepatitis A	Fatigue Malaise Anorexia Nausea/vomiting Gradual onset	Sick contacts h/o travel to endemic areas	Low grade fever RUQ pain Hepato-splenomegaly Jaundice LAD	AST/ALT Bilirubin AlkP/GGT LDH Serum IgM/IgG Anti-HAV

CC	Diagnosis	HPI	PMH	PE Findings	WorkUp
68 yo woman c/o chills, nausea, and abdominal pain	Acute cholangitis	Abd pain Jaundice Nausea/vomiting	h/o choledocholithiasis	Pt appears uncomfortable Fever RUQ pain Jaundiced	CBC w diff CRP ALT/AST/GGT Alk phosphatase Blood cultures Transabdom U/S
70 yo man c/o abdominal pain	Pancreatic cancer	Upper abd pain Unintentional weight loss Light-colored stools Dark urine Loss of appetite	Smoker h/o DM Heavy alcohol use	Jaundice FHx cancer	Abdominal CT CA 19-9 level LFT
Elderly man c/o increasing abdominal pain	Diverticulitis	Abd pain in LLQ Several days duration Gradually increasing Diarrhea and constipation	-	PT appears restless Fever LLQ tenderness Guarding Rebound	CT scan Abd x-ray CBC w/diff
65 yo man c/o bloody stools	Diverticulosis	Painless rectal bleeding Constipation Weak and fatigue Dizziness	No fiber supplements h/o HTN h/o IBS FHx of diverticulosis No FHx of colon cancer	-	Rectal exam with FOB CBC w/diff Abd x-ray Abd CT Colonoscopy
65 yo man c/o bloody stools	Colon cancer	Painless rectal bleeding Change in bowel habits Weak and fatigue Unintentional weight loss	No screening colonoscopy h/o anemia FHx of colon cancer h/o smoking	Non-specific abdominal tenderness Abdominal mass	Rectal exam with FOB CBC w/diff CT abdomen Colonoscopy
65 yo man c/o bloody stool	Angiodysplasia	Painless rectal bleeding Stool black and tarry Fatigue No weight loss No Hx of bruising	h/o anemia No FHx of colon cancer	-	Rectal exam with FOB CBC w/diff PT, PTT, INR CT abdomen Colonoscopy EGD

CC	Diagnosis	HPI	PMH	PE Findings	WorkUp
70 yo man c/o acute abdominal pain	**Mesenteric ischemia**	Acute abd. pain Pain with meals Pain out of proportion Weight loss Nausea and vomiting Blood in stool	Cardiac arrhythmia Cardiac valvular disease Infective endocarditis Recent MI Ventricular aneurysm Aortic aneurysm Aortic atherosclerosis h/o metabolic acidosis	Diffuse abd pain on palpation Abd guarding Rovsing's sign/rebound	Abd x-ray CBC ABG Lactate Abd CT angiography
Man c/o increasing abdominal pain	**Large bowel obstruction**	Severe cramping and pain Diffuse and poorly localized Abdominal distention Constipation Vomiting Unable to pass flatus	PT appears restlessness due to pain h/o prior abd. surgery	Fever Abd distention Bowel sounds normal or quiet Hyperresonance on abd. percussion Tenderness on palpation	CBC w/diff Electrolytes/anion gap Barium enema Abd x-ray Colonoscopy Abd CT scan
20 yo man c/o abdominal pain and diarrhea	**Lactose intolerance**	Bloating Diarrhea Nausea Flatulence Borborygmi Sx start 2 hrs after ingestion of lactose A/w abd cramps	h/o stomach problems	-	Hydrogen breath test Stool acidity test Fecal lactoferrin levels Calprotectin levels
20 yo man c/o abdominal pain and diarrhea	**Traveler's diarrhea**	Abd cramps Nausea Bloating Malaise Anorexia	Recent trip overseas Uses antacids for heartburn	Fever	FOB Stool culture Stool ova for parasites

CC	Diagnosis	HPI	PMH	PE Findings	WorkUp
46 yo man c/o abdominal pain and diarrhea	Crohn disease	Prolonged diarrhea w/or w/o gross bleeding Crampy abd pain Steatorrhea Aphthous ulcers or pain in mouth or gums Odynophagia Dysphagia Weight loss Fatigue Fever	FHx IBD PMh/o Eye problems (uveitis, iritis, and episcleritis) Joint problems (sacroiliitis or ankylosis spondylitis) Erythema nodosum and pyoderma gangrenosum Recurrent UTI PMh/o primary sclerosing cholangitis PMh/o pulmonary manifestations	Febrile Abd tender to palpation Abd mass	Abd x-ray Rectal exam with FOB CBC ESR and CRP PANCA and ASCA Electrolytes Colonoscopy Capsule endoscopy UGI series MRE
36 yo woman c/o abdominal pain	Irritable bowel syndrome	Diarrhea alternating with constipation A/w abd cramps Cramps alleviated by defecation Diffuse abd pain	h/o anxiety Recent exposure to excessive stress FH h/o child abuse	Generalized abd tenderness	-
46 yo man c/o abdominal pain and diarrhea	Pseudomembranous colitis	Watery diarrhea Abd pain and cramps No blood in stool	h/o allergies h/o AB therapy h/o hospitalization	Diffuse abd. tenderness to palpation	CBC w/diff Stool assay for C. difficile Rectal exam and FOB Stool for ova and parasites
30 yo woman c/o sudden onset severe abdominal pain	Appendicitis	Onset periumbilical/sharp Progressive to RLQ Anorexia/fever Nausea/vomiting Diarrhea Malaise Indigestion/flatulence	IBD	Fever Psoas/obturator sign Rovsing's sign McBurney's point tenderness	CBC w/diff Abd U/S; if neg or inconclusive then abd CT scan
40 yo woman c/o abdominal pain	Polycystic kidney disease	Headache Hematuria Polyuria	FHx of kidney disease h/o HTN h/o UTI	Hypertensive	Abd US Abd CT BUN and Creatinine

CC	Diagnosis	HPI	PMH	PE Findings	WorkUp
30 yo woman c/o sudden onset severe abdominal pain	Ectopic pregnancy	Sudden onset LLQ, RLQ pain Severe/progressive Unilateral Amenorrhea Vaginal bleeding Nausea/vomiting Breast fullness Weakness	Previous ectopic pregnancy Fallopian tube pathology and surgery Abdominal surgery In-utero DES exposure PID/infertility Uterine anomalies Smoker Progesterone/contraception/IUD	Tenderness Guarding	Pelvic exam Serum quantitative B-Hcg Transvaginal U/S
30 yo woman c/o sudden onset severe abdominal pain	PID	Lower abd pain Gradual or sudden onset Dull and achy/b/l Progressive Fever Purulent vaginal discharge Nausea/vomiting Anorexia/malaise Onset following menses	Multiple sexual partners Unprotected intercourse Bacterial vaginosis Recent gynecologic procedure HIV	Tenderness Guarding	Pelvic exam NAAT/cultures for chlamydia and gonorrhea Vaginal secretions KOH Transvaginal U/S
30 yo woman c/o sudden onset severe abdominal pain	Ovarian torsion	Sharp, intermittent, unilateral, worsening lower abdominal pain Precipitated by exercise Radiates to flank, back, and/or groin Fever Nausea/vomiting	Previously resolved episodes Pelvic surgery Ovulation induction	-	Pelvic exam Pelvic U/S Doppler
30 yo woman c/o sudden onset abdominal pain	Ovarian cyst rupture	Unilateral at onset Diffuse Exercise precipitated Vaginal bleeding Nausea/vomiting Shoulder pain	LMP 2 wks ago (midcycle)	Cullen sign	Pelvic exam Pelvic U/S Abd CT
55 yo man c/o vomiting blood	Mallory-Weiss syndrome	Vomit of bright red blood mixed with gastric content after ingesting copious amount of alcohol Light-headedness Epigastric abdominal pain	h/o smoking h/o heavy alcohol use	Pallor Diaphoretic Alcohol breath	CBC w/diff Esophagogastro-duodenoscopy

CC	Diagnosis	HPI	PMH	PE Findings	WorkUp
Middle-aged pt c/o difficulty swallowing	**Achalasia**	Progressive dysphagia to both liquids and solids A/w regurgitation of undigested food A/w chest pain behind sternum Weight loss A/w coughing when lying flat	-	Patient appears thin CV exam WNL	Esophageal manometry Barium esophagram Endoscopy
Neurology					
Young man c/o headache	**Meningitis**	Severe headache Photophobia Nuchal rigidity Fever	Rash or recent URI Recent travel	Brudzinski sign Nuchal rigidity	CBC w/diff Serum glucose Electrolytes Blood cultures/x3 CT head Lumbar puncture
Middle-aged man c/o headache	**Subarachnoid hemorrhage**	Severe headache Sudden onset Photophobia Nuchal rigidity LOC Confusion Vomiting	Recent h/o head injury	Nuchal rigidity MMSE altered	Head CT
Young woman c/o headache	**Migraine**	Unilateral headache Pulsating in nature Photophobia Visual disturbances Associated with food, menses Nausea precipitated by stress, hunger, fatigue	OCP use FHx of similar headaches	-	-
45 yo woman c/o headache	**Tension headache**	Pain in lower back of head on both sides Pain radiates to the neck Pain described as constant pressure Mild to moderate pain	Recent increased stress Sleep deprivation Recent eye strain	Tense neck and shoulder muscles	-

CC	Diagnosis	HPI	PMH	PE Findings	WorkUp
45 yo M c/o headache	Cluster headache	Unilateral orbital pain Recurrent, with periods of spontaneous remissions Severe Associated with rhinorrhea and nasal congestion No aura	Prior episodes of same headache	-	-
65 yo man c/o forgetfulness	Alzheimer disease	Progressive memory loss Confusion Impairment in occupational functioning Personality and mood changes Patient presents with progressive deterioration h/o falls Urinary incontinence Fatigue and weakness	FH of Alzheimer	MMSE Focal neurological deficits Gait disturbance	Brain MRI Brain PET scan
65 yo woman c/o forgetfulness	Vascular dementia	Cognitive deficits including memory deficits Significant impairment in social and occupational functioning Personality and mood changes, abulia, apathy Patient presents with abrupt or "step-like deterioration" h/o falls Urinary incontinence Fatigue and weakness	h/o HTN h/o strokes or cerebrovascular disease h/o high cholesterol	MMSE Focal neurological deficits Gait disturbance Hyperreflexia Babinski Pseudobulbar palsy (CN V, VII, IX, X, XI, and XII)	Brain CT and MRI
65 yo woman c/o forgetfulness and depression	Creutzfeldt-Jakob disease	Rapid progression of psychiatric Sx Depression, agitation, apathy, insomnia, irritability, social withdrawal, psychotic features (delusions and hallucinations) Dysesthesias and paresthesia on face and extremities	FHx CJD FHx psychiatric disease	Abnormal sensation Gait ataxia Involuntary movements Immobility Paresis of upward gaze Cognitive impairment Startle response and mutism	EEG Lumbar puncture Examination of tonsillar tissue Brain CT and MRI

CC	Diagnosis	HPI	PMH	PE Findings	WorkUp
65 yo man c/o vertigo	Benign positional vertigo	Episodic, each lasting a few seconds Loss of balance during episodes N/V Sudden onset Precipitated by change in head position	-	-	Dix-Hallpike test CBC w/diff CT of head Audiogram
65 yo man c/o vertigo	Cerebrovascular accident	Focal neurological deficits Symptoms >2 hrs Sudden onset	HTN DM High blood cholesterol Atrial fibrillation not compliant with warfarin FHx of early CAD h/o smoking	Focal neurological deficits	Cholesterol, HDL, LDL, triglycerides CT head Doppler U/S of carotids EKG
70 yo woman with headache and confusion	Transient ischemic attack (TIA)	Sudden onset Headache Weakness Speech disturbances and/or vision problems Duration of Sx >60 min but <24 hrs Age >60	h/o HTN h/o high cholesterol h/o DM h/o clotting dysfunction h/o MI FHx thrombotic events h/o suspected/confirmed cancer	Focal neurological deficits	Head CT Brain MRI ECG CBC w diff PT/PTT/INR Electrolytes Fasting blood lipids and glucose
70 yo woman c/o severe headache and stiff neck	Subdural hematoma	Headache Confusion Somnolence Nausea and vomiting Head trauma Falls with progressive neurological deficits development Seizures	h/o frequent falls h/o alcoholism h/o anticoagulant medication (aspirin, warfarin)	Focal neurological deficits Gait abnormalities Nuchal rigidity Brudzinski/Kernig Babinski Hemiplegia (R or L) Bruises from the falls	Head CT Brain MRI LP-CSF analysis CBC w diff PT/PTT/INR Urine toxicology

CC	Diagnosis	HPI	PMH	PE Findings	WorkUp
70 yo woman c/o severe headache and facial pain	**Trigeminal neuralgia**	Headache Sharp facial pain electric, shock- like, or stabbing Repetitive episodes (at least three) Lacrimation, conjunctival injection, and rhinorrhea Facial muscle spasm	h/o migraine h/o HTN h/o chronic facial pain h/o dull continuous pain in the jaw	No clinical evidence of neurological deficits except some sensory loss Precipitation of painful attack by tactile stimulation of facial trigger zone	Brain CT and MRI
60 yo woman c/o headache	**Temporal arteritis**	Right or Left temporal headache Tongue claudication Jaw claudication Blurred vision Acute tinnitus	Recently diagnosed with PRP	Fever Tenderness on the scalp over temporal area Jaw claudication Decreased visual acuity	ESR Biopsy of temporal artery LFT CRP Platelets
58 yo woman c/o sudden onset of back pain	**Lumbar muscle strain**	Lower back pain Sudden onset after cleaning the house Dull and achy/b/l No radiation Numbness tingling or weakness	Similar episodes in the past h/o smoking Weight gain and sedentary lifestyle During heavy work and strenuous exercise	Paraspinal tenderness and spasm No sensory deficits and motor impairments in lower extremities	L-spine x-ray L-spine MRI
58 yo woman c/o progressive onset pain in the legs	**Lumbar spinal stenosis**	Progressive onset h/o back pain and b/l leg pain Alleviated by sitting and bending forward Aggravated by walking and standing	h/o back pain h/o b/l pain in buttocks and posterior thighs FM h/o back pain	Antalgic gait Wide base gait Abnormal Romberg Vibration deficits No SLR	L-S spine x-ray L-S spine CT L-S spine MRI
58 yo man c/o numbness and tingling in his legs	**Disk herniation**	Severe back pain radiating down to buttock, leg foot and ankle Associated numbness and paresthesia Aggravated by cough, sneezing, and prolonged sitting Precipitated by lifting heavy objects Bowel and bladder Sx if b/l disk herniation	h/o back pain Occupation: carpenter h/o sciatica	Loss of sensation in L5–S1 distribution SLR ipsilateral Crossed straight leg test Loss of DTRs Impaired ankle reflex Ankle dorsiflexion weakness Great toe extensor weakness	L-S spine x-ray L-S spine CT L-S spine MRI Lower extremity EMG

CC	Diagnosis	HPI	PMH	PE Findings	WorkUp
35 yo woman c/o numbness and tingling in her legs	Multiple sclerosis	Varying degree of relapsing remitting sensory weakness and visual disturbances Pain, light touch, and proprioceptive loss Bilateral sensory loss in limb and face from a certain level down Vertigo Fatigue Urinary incontinence Heat sensitivity Gait disturbance, incoordination, balance problems Headache Painful spasms	h/o epilepsy h/o anxiety, depression, and cognitive impairment h/o anemia h/o sleep disorders and sleep apnea h/o Cr. thyroid disorders and infections h/o mobility limitations h/o trigeminal neuralgia h/o back pain h/o restless leg syndrome	Weaknesses associated with spasticity, hyperreflexia, and clonus Lhermitte phenomenon Monocular vison/visual field loss (scotoma) and difficulty discerning color Marcus Gunn pupils Internuclear ophthalmoplegia Horizontal nystagmus Spastic paraparesis Limb ataxias	Brain MRI Spinal MRI CS analysis for oligo-clonal bands Visual evoked potential Somatosensory evoked potential
55 yo man c/o numbness in his hands and feet	Diabetic peripheral neuropathy	Numbness and tingling in hands and feet for few mos Pain in the legs Duration ≥6 mo Constipation Impotence Vision problems	h/o DM h/o alcoholism h/o HTN h/o otitis media	Decreased soft, vibratory, and positions sense Sores on feet	Glucose level HbA1C Nerve conduction study EMG
66 yo man c/o forgetfulness	Parkinson disease	Feeling slow in processing information and thinking for last few months Loss of dexterity (noted when dressing) Slight tremor in right hand Malaise Sleep disturbances Decreased sense of smell Slow in movement (bradykinesia) Constipation	Occupation: farmer	Soft spoken, slow speech Masked facies (hypomimia) Resting tremor Bradykinesia Rigidity	
30 yo woman c/o headache	Idiopathic intracranial hypertension	Throbbing headache Headache worse in the morning and worse with coughing/sneezing Nausea/vomiting Pulsatile tinnitus Double vision	Used isotretinoin for acne	CNS examination Fundoscopy Obese	Brain CT Lumbar puncture w/CSF analysis

CC	Diagnosis	HPI	PMH	PE Findings	WorkUp
Musculoskeletal					
35 yo woman c/o pain in left hand	**Carpal tunnel syndrome**	Pain in last 3 digits of left hand and wrist Numbness and tingling Pain radiated up forearm	Occupation involves repetitive movement h/o hypothyroidism Multiple pregnancies	Tenderness to palpation of first digits and wrist Decreased muscle strength in left hand Decreased sensation in first 3 digits of left hand Phalen or Tinel sign positive	Nerve conduction study EMG Left hand and wrist x-ray
Middle-aged woman c/o joint pain	**Rheumatoid arthritis**	Symmetric morning stiffness >1h Duration 6 wks Improved w/motion Swelling of the hands Low-grade fever Fatigue for several mos	FHx of RA	Rheumatoid nodules Decreased ROM on hands and fingers Tender joints with ROM	Anti-cyclic citrullinated peptide ANA, RF Hand/wrist x-ray
Middle-aged woman c/o joint pain	**SLE**	Morning stiffness <1hr Photosensitivity Oral ulcers Alopecia Weight loss Swelling and redness of affected joints Fatigue	FH of immune disease	Malar/discoid rash Low grade fever Petechiae Decreased ROM on affected joints Tender joints with ROM	ANA Anti-dsDNA AB Anti-Sm AB Complement level Antiphospholipid antibodies INR
Middle-aged woman c/o joint pain	**Lyme disease**	Erythema migrans rash Arthralgias/myalgias Onset: migratory, polyarticular Progression: monoarticular h/o tick bite Lives in Northeast, mid-Atlantic, or upper Midwest Swelling and redness of affected joints Fatigue	Hx of tick bite or walking in the woods	Bell palsy Bradycardia Heart block Target rash will not be present at this stage Low-grade fever Decreased ROM on affected joints Tender joints with ROM	Lyme titer: ELISA/Western blot
Middle-aged woman c/o pain in left hip	**Osteoarthritis**	Morning stiffness <30 min Monoarticular/polyarticular Asymmetric Insidious progression Aggravated by exercise Relieved by rest	FH Obesity Trauma/repetitive stress Previous surgery	< ROM	Hip x-ray

CC	Diagnosis	HPI	PMH	PE Findings	WorkUp
Middle-aged woman c/o pain in left hip	**Polymyalgia rheumatica**	Morning stiffness >30 min Distal extremities Fatigue Anorexia/weight loss Fever Headaches Scalp tenderness	Carpal tunnel syndrome Temporal arteritis	PIP affected Nodules	ESR CRP MRI or U/S of involved joints
Middle-aged woman c/o pain in left hip	**Multiple myeloma**	Bone pain: spine, long bones, skull, pelvis, chest Severe/intermittent Aggravated by movement Relieved by rest Fatigue/generalized weakness Weight loss	Anemia Recent bacterial infection	Back pain	Serum protein electrophoresis U/A Bence Jones proteins & albumin Peripheral smear Skeletal survey Serum Ca
45 yo man c/o worsening joint pain and morning stiffness	**Psoriatic arthritis**	Joint pain with polyarthritis Asymmetric arthritis affecting multiple joints (Oligoarthritis) Morning stiffness >30 min Aggravated by prolonged immobility Alleviated by physical exercise Back pain h/o skin disease	FHx psoriasis FHx RA h/o spondyloarthritis: sacroiliitis and spondylitis h/o enthesitis and tenosynovitis h/o arthritis mutilans h/o CV diseases or stroke h/o Achilles tendinitis and plantar fasciitis h/o gout	Stress pain, joint line tenderness and effusion in affected joint DIP joints pain and deformity Sausage digits Decreased ROM in affected joints Dactylitis Skin lesions especially at joint pressure points Nail pitting, onycholysis Hyperkeratosis Splinter hemorrhages Pitting edema Conjunctivitis and uveitis	CBC ESR and CRP RF ANA Anti-CCP antibodies HLA B-27 HLA-C*06 x-ray and MRI of affected joint Arthrocentesis and synovial fluid analysis BUN/uric acid/U/A
Patient c/o pain in left foot	**Gout**	Acute onset Swelling of ankle joint Monoarticular or oligoarticular Asymmetric Increased from foods with purines Increased with exercise Low-grade fever	Prior episode Trauma/diuretics Alcohol h/o nephrolithiasis Metabolic syndrome	Podagra Erythema	Joint aspiration with synovial fluid analysis Angle x-ray for crystal Uric acid level in blood

CC	Diagnosis	HPI	PMH	PE Findings	WorkUp
45 yo man with worsening joint pain and morning stiffness	Disseminated gonococcal infection	C/o tenosynovitis Asymmetric mono or polyarthralgia Dermatitis Fever, chills Generalized malaise h/o multiple sexual partners Unprotected intercourse	h/o congenital or acquired complement deficiency h/o SLE h/o STI	Purulent arthritis Pustular or vesiculo-pustular dermatitis Tenosynovitis with redness and warmth around tendon sheath	CBC w/diff Blood culture on Thayer-Martin media PCR for Gonococcal DNA Synovial fluid analysis from affected joints Skin lesion specimens
45 yo man c/o worsening joint pain	Lateral epicondylitis	Elbow pain, swelling, and loss of motion Repetitive elbow movement Numbness and tingling in the hand h/o cervical neck pain	h/o trauma h/o smoking h/o gout h/o gonorrhea h/o IBS	Local tenderness, swelling, and redness at affected joint Impaired ROM Sensory loss	CXR x-ray and MRI of affected joint Arthrocentesis CBC Uric acid level
43 yo woman c/o hip pain	Hip dislocation	h/o recent fall	Long-term smoker Recent hip replacement surgery	Tenderness on palpation of hip Limited ROM of hip	Hip x-ray MRI of affected hip
82 yo woman c/o inability to bear weight	Hip fracture	Recent fall Hip pain	PMH of osteoporosis	Tenderness to palpation of hip	Hip x-ray MRI of affected hip
45 yo woman c/o muscle weakness	Myasthenia gravis	Weakness worse at night and with exertion Weakness alleviated with rest Diplopia Difficulty chewing and swallowing Slurred speech Droopy eyelids Progressive fatigue Jaw weakness with chewing Difficulty walking up-stairs No muscle pain	FHx of hypothyroidism and RA	Slurred speech Drooping eyelids Decreased muscle strength Decreased reflexes in UE and LE b/l	Acetylcholine receptor antibodies Muscle specific tyrosine kinase antibodies Anti-striated muscle antibodies (anti-SM) EMG, NCS
45 yo man c/o muscle weakness	Guillain-Barre syndrome	Ascending symmetrical weakness Numbness and tingling Progressive fatigue Diplopia Slurred speech	Recent URI	Low BP and high HR Eyes: ptosis Loss of deep tendon reflexes in LE b/l Decreased muscle strength in LE b/l	EMG, NCS FVC, negative inspiratory force (NIF)

CC	Diagnosis	HPI	PMH	PE Findings	WorkUp
Patient c/o pain in left lower leg	Cellulitis	Ankle area extending up LLE +/– puncture wound Swelling/erythema/ unilateral Fever/chills/malaise No drainage	Trauma few days prior Skin disorder at site DM/HIV Surgery	Lymph nodes Erythema	CBC w/diff
Patient c/o pain in left lower leg	Peripheral artery disease (PAD)	Worse with ambulation Worse when climbing stairs Alleviated when exertion stops Intermittent/cramping/ claudication	h/o hyperlipidemia/ DM/MI h/o HTN Smoker FHx	Diminished/absent pulses Shiny skin/absent hair Cold feet Thickened toenails Impaired sensation	Ankle/brachial arterial pressure index Duplex U/S
57 yo woman c/o significant pain and swelling of her left leg for past several days	Deep vein thrombosis (DVT)	Pain w/leg Leg swelling (circumference ≥3cm in affected leg compared to non-affected) OCPs and smoking Sedentary lifestyle Dyspnea of sudden onset/ chest pain/fatigue if complicated with PE	Malignancy h/o prior DVT h/o immobilization >3 days h/o surgery >30 min Pregnancy Estrogen therapy Smoking Obesity h/o venous thrombo- embolism	Localized tenderness Entire leg swollen Pitting edema in symptomatic leg Collateral superficial veins (non-varicose) in affected LE Increased warmth at affected side Tachypnea	Doppler U/S of LE D-dimers CTA Antiphospholipid ABies Factor V Leiden Prot C and S INR, TTP, PT Homocysteine level Antithrombin III and Fct VIII CXR ABG ECG
50 yo man c/o pain in heel and bottom of foot	Plantar fasciitis	Sharp unilateral pain Worse at periods of rest and in morning	h/o smoking Runner	Obese Pain reproduced by bending foot and toes up toward the shin	-
45 yo man c/o gradual onset of localized chest pain	Costochondritis	Regional pain syndrome Stinging pain Pain reproducible by palpation Multiple areas of chest tenderness Absence of cough	No significant PMH	Tenderness at upper costal cartilage of costochondral or costosternal junctions Localized muscle tension No heat erythema or localized swelling	CXR

CC	Diagnosis	HPI	PMH	PE Findings	WorkUp
Psychiatry					
Patient c/o dizziness	Panic disorder	Unexpected episodes of palpitations, SOB, dizziness Associated w/sweating, trembling, chest pain, palpitations and circumoral numbness Persistent concern about future attacks	H/x of anxiety No h/x of substance abuse FHx of caffeine use	-	-
Patient c/o dizziness	Acute alcohol intoxication	Dizziness Euphoria Ataxia Slurred speech Vomiting Confusion	H/x alcohol abuse FHx of alcoholism Stressful job	Alcohol scent on breath Gait unstable Slurred speech MMSE	Serum ethanol level Urine toxicology Serum glucose level
25 yo man c/o visual hallucinations	Substance-induced psychosis	Disorientation Acute intoxication of alcohol	Alcoholic Cannabis use	-	Urine toxicology
23 yo man c/o restlessness	Schizophrenia	h/o >6 mo of delusion, hallucinations (auditory), social dysfunction, and disorganized speech Interferes with normal functioning	FH	MMSE Impaired judgment Blunt affect	Urine tox screen Head CT Brain MRI Brain PET scan
18 yo man c/o difficulty concentrating	Schizoaffective disorder	Delusions Hallucinations Alogia Avolition Anhedonia Irritable mood Excessive agitation	h/o anxiety Risk taking behavior	Disorganized speech Blunt affect	CBC w/diff Electrolytes Serum glucose Cortisol Urine tox screen Serum alcohol level TSH

CC	Diagnosis	HPI	PMH	PE Findings	WorkUp
25 yo woman c/o fatigue	Bipolar disorder	Sad mood >2 wks Early morning wakefulness Anhedonia Loss of concentration Decreased appetite Suicidal ideations Associated with periods of increased energy, excessive spending, and increased promiscuous sexual activity	FHx of similar symptoms	Affect depressed Mood c/w affect	CBC w/diff Electrolytes Serum glucose Cortisol Urine tox screen Serum alcohol level TSH
20 yo woman c/o depressed mood	Adjustment disorder	Loss of interest Feeling of hopelessness Alleviated with removal of stressor Sadness Anhedonia Difficulty concentrating	Loss of job 1 mo ago	Depressed affect Affect c/w mood	CBC w/diff Electrolytes Serum glucose Cortisol Urine tox screen Serum alcohol level TSH
25 yo woman c/o fatigue	Major depressive disorder	Sad mood >2 wks Early morning wakefulness Anhedonia Loss of concentration Decreased appetite Suicidal ideations	FHx of psychiatric conditions	Decreased concentration on MMSE Depressed affect Mood c/w affect Lack of eye contact	CBC w/diff Electrolytes Serum glucose Cortisol Urine tox screen Serum alcohol level TSH
35 yo woman c/o fatigue	Normal bereavement	Anhedonia Anorexia Trouble concentrating Trouble sleeping	Loss of husband 6 mos ago	-	-
20 yo woman c/o fatigue	Social Anxiety Disorder (Social Phobia)	Persistent fear of one or more social or performance situations h/o of diaphoresis, tremors, palpitations, and nausea in public places Avoidance of public spaces	h/o anxiety	Anxious mood Mood c/w affect	CBC w/diff Electrolytes Serum glucose Cortisol Urine tox screen Serum alcohol level TSH

CC	Diagnosis	HPI	PMH	PE Findings	WorkUp
Pediatrics					
Mother c/o child becoming irritable lately	Lead poisoning	Anorexia (picky eater) Abd pain/constipation Poor attention span Distractibility Impulsiveness/ hyperactivity Pica/lethargy Vomiting/headache	Lives in old building Low socioeconomic status	-	Physical exam Blood lead level CBC
Mother c/o child becoming irritable lately	Iron deficiency anemia	Anorexia (picky eater) Lethargy Fatigue Pallor Irritability Poor feeding Pica Diet mainly of milk	Low birth weight Blood loss Systolic murmur	-	Physical exam Peripheral smear Serum iron/ ferritin TIBC/FEP Reticulocyte count FOB CBC/MCV/RDW
Mother c/o child becoming irritable lately	**Attention deficit hyperactivity disorder (ADHD)**	Inattention/hyperactivity Impulsivity Multiple settings Onset age <12 Duration ≥6 mos Distracted/disorganized Forgetful Constant fidgeting Short attention span Tasks not completed	FH Psychiatric disorder	-	Physical examination Psychiatric mental status evaluation
Parent c/o 7 yo child with irritability	**Oppositional defiant disorder**	Patterns of argumentative behavior Symptoms ≥6 mos Often loses temper/angry Argues with authority figures Deliberately annoys classmates Blames others for his mistakes	-	-	Physical exam

CC	Diagnosis	HPI	PMH	PE Findings	WorkUp
Mother c/o child with fever and rash	Measles	Cough, coryza, and conjunctivitis h/o recent travel or exposure to sick persons Transient respiratory Sx Fever Malaise, anorexia Diarrhea Lethargy	h/o otitis media Missed vaccinations	Fever Maculopapular rash Koplik spots Keratitis or corneal ulcerations Non-purulent conjunctivitis LAD	Physical examination Serum measles IgM and IgG antibodies RT-PCR for measles virus RNA CBC w/diff
Mother c/o newborn with fever and lethargy	Neonatal sepsis	Fever Lethargy Poor feeding Poor tone Irritability Seizures	h/o inherited metabolic disorders Hypoxia Acidosis GBS infection h/o maternal chorioamnionitis Intrapartum-fetal tachycardia APGAR <6 Meconium ileus	Respiratory distress: tachypnea, flaring, grunting, and use of respiratory muscles Tachycardia Hypotension Fever	Physical examination CBC w/diff CRP Blood cultures LP CXR (if respiratory distress)
Mother c/o newborn with irritability and crying	Colic	Irritability Paroxysmal crying especially in the evening Relieved by flatus or bowel movement Normal feeding	-	Face of baby is flushed Distended and tensed abdomen Clenched fingers Stiff and extended arms Arched back Otherwise NL PE	Bring child for PE
Mother c/o newborn who is irritable and cries inconsolably	Intussusception	Progressive intermittent cramping Sudden severe abd pain at 15-20 min intervals Inconsolable cry Bilious emesis Lethargy Altered consciousness	h/o reactive lymphoid hyperplasia h/o gastroenteritis FHx GI problems: Meckel, Crohn, celiac, cystic fibrosis	Child is drawing his legs up toward the abdomen Abd distension Palpable sausage-shaped abd mass	Bring child for PE FOB for gross blood and currant jelly stool Abd U/S Abd plain x-ray
Mother c/o newborn unable to pass stool	Hirschsprung disease	A/w brown vomit Abd swelling Flatulence	-	-	Physical exam

CC	Diagnosis	HPI	PMH	PE Findings	WorkUp
16 yo girl c/o cold intolerance	**Anorexia nervosa**	Weight loss Food restriction Excessive exercise	Use of laxatives Amenorrhea Brittle hair Fatigue Fhx of eating disorders	Thin appearance Lanugo Hypotensive	Electrolytes CBC
Fatigue					
Patient c/o fatigue	Hypothyroidism	Weight (gain) Cold intolerance/dry skin Brittle hair/puffy face/ sleepiness Constipation Depressed mood Muscle weakness Decreased sweating Hoarseness Lower extremity edema Impaired memory Tongue enlargement	Potential drug-induced: lithium Hypothalamic-pituitary axis damage Menstrual abnormalities Carpal tunnel syndrome h/o Autoimmune disease FHx of hypothyroidism	Loss of eyebrows/ periorbital edema Deep tendon reflexes: delayed relaxation Edema	TSH Free T4
Patient c/o fatigue	**B12 deficiency**	Weight loss Decreased appetite Unsteady gait Numbness/tingling of feet and hands Perception of wearing stockings or gloves Constipation or diarrhea Sore tongue/weakness Psychosis/memory loss Pallor Palpitations/DOE	Vegan diet Alcoholic Pernicious anemia Crohn disease/celiac sprue GI resection Acid-suppressing drugs Metformin Bacterial overgrowth	Extremities: MRS Romberg sign Altered gait	CBC Serum B12 level Methylmalonic acid/ homocysteine level Peripheral smear
Patient c/o fatigue	**Iron deficiency anemia**	Angular cheilitis Pica Lethargy/pallor Palpitations/DOE Poor exercise tolerance Lightheadedness/leg cramps Glossitis/koilonychia	GI bleed/ menorrhagia/celiac sprue Recent infections Bacterial overgrowth Systolic murmur	Pallor Tachycardia	Peripheral smear Serum iron/ ferritin TIBC/CBC

CC	Diagnosis	HPI	PMH	PE Findings	WorkUp
Patient c/o fatigue	**Non-Hodgkin lymphoma**	Fever/night sweats/weight loss Skin rash, pruritus Anorexia/weight loss Nausea/vomiting Cr. pain, abd fullness, early satiety Headache Lethargy Seizures	PMHx/FHx lymphoma or hematopoietic malignancy h/o radiation or chemotherapy Exposure to agricultural pesticides and hair dyes	Painless, peripheral lymphadenopathy Hepatosplenomegaly Fever of unknown etiology Focal neurological deficits	CBC w/diff Serum LDH and uric acid Serum Ca level Peripheral smear Serum protein electrophoresis CXR CT abd PET/CT brain LN biopsy
35 yo woman c/o fatigue	**Post-traumatic stress disorder (PTSD)**	Flashbacks Nightmares Sxs persist >1 mo post-trauma	Recent major trauma	-	-
Personal Problems					
67 yo man with personal problem	**Drug-related erectile dysfunction**	h/o erectile dysfunction Non-compliant with HTA and DM medication	h/o HTN h/o MI h/o DM h/o radical prostatectomy	Abn peripheral sensation on LE Abn femoral/peripheral pulses Alopecia, gynecomastia Visual field defects	Genital examination Nocturnal penile tumescence test MRI brain Glucose level and HbA1C Testosterone and prolactin levels Duplex Doppler imaging of penis Lipid profile
DM Follow Up					
Patient c/o tremor palpitations and anxiety	**Diabetes Mellitus**	Polyuria, polydipsia, polyphagia h/o hypoglycemic Sx Weight gain (or weight loss if DM I) Sedentary lifestyle High fat diet History of claudication	h/o CV disease h/o HTN h/o high Cholesterol h/o PAD h/o obesity h/o smoking	Obese patient Peripheral pulses diminished in LE Sensation impaired in LE	Blood glucose level HbA1C Fasting lipid profile Urine albumin AST/ALT Serum creatinine TSH (if type I DM)

CC	Diagnosis	HPI	PMH	PE Findings	WorkUp
Domestic Violence					
41 yo woman c/o insomnia	**Domestic violence**	h/o abd pain Depressed mood Difficulty falling asleep Pain on bruised area Abd pain or others Sx	h/o depression h/o visiting the clinic multiple times w/o a clear dg	Bruises Inspection of other skin or body parts with traces of trauma in different stages of healing	X-ray skeletal survey FAST U/S for soft tissue trauma
Sleep Disorders					
41 yo woman c/o insomnia	**Stress induced insomnia**	Difficulty falling asleep and staying asleep Anxiety Fatigue Constant unreasonable worries and tension Impaired daytime function Inability to concentrate Weight loss or gain Memory problems h/o multiple coffee/day	FHX of bipolar disorder or other psychiatric disorder h/o starting new medication (e.g., SSRI) h/o anxiety disorders Pt undergoing a very stressful situation (domestic violence, stress at work/home, etc.) h/o Ac/Cr pain or permanent disability h/o using recreational drugs and alcohol	NL thyroid examination DTR's intact b/l Motor 5/5 b/l	CBC TSH, T3, T4 U/Tox
35 yo man c/o fatigue	**Obstructive sleep apnea**	Snoring Morning headaches Excessive daytime sleepiness	Smoker	Obese Hypertensive	Polysomnography
Miscellaneous					
19 yo woman c/o frequent nose bleeds	von Willebrand disease	Copious nosebleed that lasted >35 min Aspirin use after mild headache	h/o easy bruising h/o 1 episode of heavy bleeding after tooth extraction h/o menorrhagia FHx of bleeding disorder	Epistaxis arising from Little's area Bruising in lower extremity	PT/aPTT Factor VIII Ristocetin cofactor
24 yo woman c/o itching and a rash	Drug-induced urticaria	Sudden onset of generalized intense itching of 3 hrs duration Appearance of a rash that started on chest and back and then spread to abdomen and extremities	h/o tonsillitis 2 days ago; currently being treated with amoxicillin	Circular blanchable, raised wheals in chest, abdomen, and extremities	-

PART V

Putting It All Together

Putting It All Together: CIS, SEP, and ICE

8

The following 31 cases are designed to give you additional practice with Step 2 CS–style scenarios. They should be used after you have reviewed all of the earlier chapters in this book. Remember, when you take the CS exam, you'll need to pass all 3 components in order to get an overall passing score.

Depending on your individual strengths and weaknesses, you can select how to best use these cases to your advantage.

Option 1: If you need practice on all 3 components: CIS, SEP, and ICE

Practice these cases with a study partner. Play the "role" of the doctor (don't read the case before your study session).

- Your study partner will play the role of the patient (he/she will need to review the case prior to the study session to answer the questions appropriately).
- Set a timer for 15 minutes before you start.
- Read the "doorway information" and write down the necessary information on a scrap sheet of paper (mnemonics and a differential diagnosis for the chief complaint).
- Knock on the door, introduce yourself, and start on the focused history/focused physical exam on the "patient" (your study partner).
- Assess your ability to identify the CIS sub-components using the checklist for the case.
- If English is not your first language, practice the common phrases reviewed in this book.
- Your study partner can also mark the information you are able to elicit from the history. Review the checklist afterward and think about what questions you should have asked. Remember, there is no history checklist on the exam; this is simply a tool to assist your preparation for the exam.
- The physical exam checklist provides a suggested focused physical exam for each case. Your study partner should share with you as many of the findings as possible.

After the 15 minutes is over, reset your timer for 10 minutes and type a Patient Note. **Use the Patient Note template** available at **usmle.org/practice-materials**. The most efficient way to improve your Patient Notes is to practice using the USMLE template, and type lots and lots of notes!

After completing the steps, grade your own Patient Notes using the provided samples. Have your study partner grade CIS, SEP, and the physical examination components of ICE using the appropriate checklists.

Option 2: If you need practice only with writing the Patient Note

As you review each case, use the margins as you would use scrap paper on the exam to write down any important findings.

- Begin to draw a mental picture of the patient and the differential diagnosis.
- Predict what you think the relevant history and physical exam items would be.
- Type a Patient Note using the USMLE template, including the significant positives and negatives from the history and physical exam.
- Indicate your list of differential diagnoses with justifications and diagnostic workup plans.

Review your predictions and notes with the answers found in the **Patient Notes** that follow.

CASE 1: FATIGUE, COUGH, AND CHEST PAIN

Doorway Information

Opening Scenario

Daniel Johnson, a 52-year-old man, presents with fatigue and cough for the past 6 months, and chest pain for the past 2 days.

Vital Signs

T 38.2 C (100.8 F)

BP 132/90 mm Hg

Pulse 91/min

Respirations 22/min

Pulse oximetry 92% on room air

Examinee Tasks

1. Obtain a focused history.

2. Perform a relevant physical exam. Do not perform rectal, pelvic, genitourinary, or corneal reflex exam.

3. Discuss your initial diagnostic impression and your workup plan with the patient.

4. After leaving the room, complete your Patient Note.

Communication and Interpersonal Skills Checklist

Fostering the Relationship	Gathering Information	Providing Information
☐ Knocked ☐ Introduced self ☐ Clarified role ☐ Was properly groomed ☐ Made eye contact ☐ Maintained appropriate distance ☐ Displayed confident manner ☐ Showed care and concern ☐ Was respectful and nonjudgmental ☐ Established patient's preferred title ☐ Used proper draping ☐ Focused on patient ☐ Did not interrupt patient ☐ Maintained appropriate and responsive body language	☐ Elicited chief complaint ☐ Established timeline of patient's CC ☐ Used open-ended question ☐ Used non-leading questions ☐ Used closed-ended questions ☐ Asked one question at a time ☐ Did not use medical jargon ☐ Appropriately used "continuers" ☐ Paraphrased ☐ Appropriately used transitions ☐ Elicited additional concerns ☐ Assessed impact on patient's life ☐ Checked for patient understanding	☐ Summarized significant information ☐ Provided diagnostic impression ☐ Justified diagnosis with evidence from encounter ☐ Assessed patient's need for additional information ☐ Encouraged and answered questions ☐ Assessed patient's comprehension of probable illness

Making Decisions	Supporting Emotions
☐ Clearly stated next steps in management ☐ Counseled patient ☐ Agreed to mutual plan of action	☐ Actively listened and validated patient's expectations ☐ Showed empathy and used appropriate reassurances ☐ Inquired about patient's support system ☐ Managed the challenge (here; patient asked, "Is it serious?")

History and Physical Examination Checklist

HPI

- ☐ Worsening cough
  - ☐ Duration: 6 Months
  - ☐ Productive and hacking
- ☐ Sputum
  - ☐ Blood tinged
  - ☐ Rusty colored
  - ☐ Small quantity
- ☐ Night sweats
- ☐ Low grade fever
- ☐ Fatigue
- ☐ Chest pain
  - ☐ Right sided
  - ☐ Sharp
  - ☐ Worse when he breathes deeply
  - ☐ Started a few days ago
  - ☐ Pain 4/10
  - ☐ No radiation
- ☐ Improves with cough suppressants and OTC acetaminophen
- ☐ No orthopnea or SOB
- ☐ No wasting or malaise
- ☐ 20 lb weight loss
  - ☐ Over the last 4 months
  - ☐ Doesn't feel hungry

PMH

- ☐ No similar illness
- ☐ History of previous recurrent pneumonia
  - ☐ Treated
  - ☐ Did not make follow up visits
- ☐ No hospitalizations or surgery
- ☐ Meds: no prescription meds
- ☐ OTC: acetaminophen, cough suppressants
- ☐ NKDA

Family Hx

- ☐ No significant family history
- ☐ Not been around anyone sick recently

Social Hx

- ☐ Recently released from prison
- ☐ Longtime cellmate with serious cough
- ☐ History of sex with men
- ☐ Unsure of HIV status
- ☐ Inconsistent condom use
- ☐ Heroin use
- ☐ Smokes 1–2 packs per day
- ☐ No alcohol use

Physical Examination

- ☐ Washed hands prior to examination
- ☐ Inspected oropharynx
- ☐ Palpated neck/supraclavicular area for lymphadenopathy
- ☐ Palpated chest for tactile fremitus
  - ☐ Decreased tactile vocal fremitus bilaterally
- ☐ Palpated chest wall for tenderness
- ☐ Percussed lungs posteriorly bilaterally
- ☐ Percussed lungs anteriorly bilaterally
- ☐ Auscultated lungs posteriorly bilaterally
  - ☐ Few bibasilar rales
- ☐ Auscultated lungs anteriorly bilaterally
  - ☐ Few bibasilar rales
- ☐ Auscultated heart (4 areas: A, P, T, M)
- ☐ Examined extremities for clubbing, cyanosis, and/or edema

Patient Note

History

CC: 52 yo M c/o fatigue and cough for the past 6 months and chest pain for the past 2 days.

HPI: cough getting progressively worse, a/w occasional small amounts of blood-tinged sputum (rusty-colored), + fatigue, + night sweats, + low grade fevers, + sharp, pleuritic right sided chest pain (4/10, does not radiate) × 2d, + 20 lb weight loss / 4 mos, + anorexia, no orthopnea, no acute SOB

ROS: denies abdominal pain, nausea, vomiting, wasting, malaise, retrosternal or interscapular chest pain, arthralgia and chills

PMH: several episodes of "pneumonia"

Meds: occasional acetaminophen and OTC cough suppressants

Social hx: 1-2 ppd of cigarettes, + heroin use, no ETOH, recently released from prison

Sexual hx: sexually active with men, HIV and other STD status unknown, denies recent travel or sick contacts

---

Physical Examination

T 100.8 F, respirations 22/min, pulse 91/min, BP 132/90 mm Hg

Pulse oximetry 92% on room air

General: In moderate respiratory distress, but cooperative

HEENT: Oropharynx - no erythema, exudates, ulcers, or thrush. No LAD.

Chest: bibasilar rales and decreased tactile fremitus bilaterally

Cough on expiration, pleuritic pain on right with deep inspiration

Clear to percussion. No chest wall tenderness

CV: Sl/S2 WNL, RRR, no M/R/G

Ext: no edema, clubbing, or cyanosis

Data Interpretation

DIAGNOSIS 1. PULMONARY TUBERCULOSIS

History Findings	Physical Exam Findings
6 month cough	Fever and tachypnea
Hemoptysis	Moderate respiratory distress
Night sweats	Pleuritic pain on right
Low-grade fever	Cough on expiration
Fatigue	Rales and decreased tactile fremitus bilaterally
Sharp, pleuritic right-sided chest pain	Pulse oximetry 92% on room air
Decreased appetite (20 lbs. weight loss/4 mos)	
Recent prison release	

DIAGNOSIS 2. PNEUMOCYSTIS JIROVECI PNEUMONIA

History Findings	Physical Exam Findings
6 month cough	Fever and tachypnea
Hemoptysis	Moderate respiratory distress
Low-grade fever	Pleuritic pain on right
History of sex with men	Pulse oximetry 92% on room air
Unknown HIV status	
Sharp, pleuritic right-sided chest pain	
Weight loss and decreased appetite	
Fatigue	

Diagnostic Studies

CBC w/differential

CXR PA and lateral

Sputum for Gram stain and culture

QuantiFERON-TB Gold (QFT-G) test

PPD with controls

HIV RNA PCR

Case Tips and Possible Alternatives

Critical Findings	Case Variations DDX	Important to Communicate
☐ Cough >6 months ☐ Hemoptysis ☐ Fatigue, night sweats, fever ☐ Weight loss ☐ Prison ☐ Sex with men ☐ Unknown HIV status	☐ Lung cancer (cigarette smoking + weight loss) ☐ Histoplasmosis (unknown HIV status) ☐ Lung abscess (Hx. of alcoholism + deficient oral care)	☐ Check HIV status ☐ Practicing safe sex ☐ Tobacco cessation ☐ Adapting to life after prison
Note: Asking patients length of stay in prison, conditions of the prison environment, and reason for stay can give reveal important information that can guide further questions, approach, and counseling.		

CASE 2: BACK PAIN AND FEVER

Doorway Information

Opening Scenario

Jane Williams is a 63-year-old woman who presents with back pain and fever for the past 3 days.

Vital Signs

T 38.3 C (101.0 F)

BP 129/85 mm Hg

Pulse 108/min

Respirations 16/min

Examinee Tasks

1. Obtain a focused history.

2. Perform a relevant physical exam. Do not perform rectal, pelvic, genitourinary, female breast, or corneal reflex exam.

3. Discuss your initial diagnostic impression and your workup plan with the patient.

4. After leaving the room, complete your Patient Note.

Communication and Interpersonal Skills Checklist

Fostering the Relationship	Gathering Information	Providing Information
☐ Knocked	☐ Elicited chief complaint	☐ Summarized significant information
☐ Introduced self	☐ Established timeline of patient's CC	☐ Provided diagnostic impression
☐ Clarified role	☐ Used open-ended question	☐ Justified diagnosis with evidence from encounter
☐ Was properly groomed	☐ Used non-leading questions	
☐ Made eye contact	☐ Used closed-ended questions	☐ Assessed patient's need for additional information
☐ Maintained appropriate distance	☐ Asked one question at a time	
☐ Displayed confident manner	☐ Did not use medical jargon	☐ Encouraged and answered questions
☐ Showed care and concern	☐ Appropriately used "continuers"	
☐ Was respectful and nonjudgmental	☐ Paraphrased	☐ Assessed patient's comprehension of probable illness
☐ Established patient's preferred title	☐ Appropriately used transitions	
☐ Used proper draping	☐ Elicited additional concerns	
☐ Focused on patient	☐ Assessed impact on patient's life	
☐ Did not interrupt patient	☐ Checked for patient understanding	
☐ Maintained appropriate and responsive body language		

Making Decisions	Supporting Emotions
☐ Clearly stated next steps in management	☐ Actively listened and validated patient's expectations
☐ **Counseled** patient	☐ Showed empathy and used appropriate reassurances
☐ Agreed to **mutual plan** of action	☐ Inquired about patient's support system
	☐ Managed the **challenge** (here; patient asked, "Can I have something for the pain?")

History and Physical Examination Checklist

HPI

- ☐ Nausea and fatigue
- ☐ Duration: 3 days
- ☐ Patient assumed it was flu initially
- ☐ Progressively felt worse
- ☐ Back pain
  - ☐ Mid to lower, right side pain
  - ☐ Dull 5/10 intensity
  - ☐ Constant
  - ☐ Radiates to groin
- ☐ Increased urinary frequency
- ☐ + burning during urination
- ☐ No blood in urine or discoloration
- ☐ + fever
- ☐ + chills
- ☐ Fever alleviated by acetaminophen

Denies:

- ☐ Vomiting, constipation, diarrhea
- ☐ SOB or headache
- ☐ Pelvic or perineal pain
- ☐ Numbness or tingling LE
- ☐ No other aggravating or alleviating factors

PMH

- ☐ Recurrent urinary tract infections
- ☐ Last episode 1 year ago
- ☐ No history of kidney stones
- ☐ History of diabetes mellitus type 2
- ☐ Diabetic foot ulcer
- ☐ Recent HgA1c 6.8%
- ☐ HTN
- ☐ Meds: metformin, lisinopril, and acetaminophen
- ☐ NKDA

Family Hx

- ☐ No relevant family history

Social Hx

- ☐ No alcohol, no drugs
- ☐ No tobacco use
  - ☐ LMP 11 years ago
  - ☐ Pap smear 3 years ago
  - ☐ G2P2
  - ☐ Sexually active w/husband
  - ☐ No recent travel

Physical Examination

- ☐ Washed hands prior to examination
- ☐ Inspected abdomen
- ☐ Auscultated abdomen in 4 quadrants
- ☐ Percussed abdomen in 4 quadrants
- ☐ Palpated abdomen in 4 quadrants
- ☐ Examined for costovertebral angle tenderness (CVAT)
  - ☐ Positive
- ☐ Palpated lumbosacral spine and paraspinal muscles
- ☐ Performed straight leg raise test
- ☐ Examined extremities
  - ☐ Ulceration on plantar surface

Patient Note

History

CC: 63 yo F c/o back pain and fever for the past 3 days.

HPI: Right-sided pain of her mid to lower back associated with nausea and fatigue. She thought she had the flu and stayed in bed with plenty of fluids and rest. A day later, the chills and fever started. She describes the pain as dull and constant, with radiation to the groin. Pain is 5/10. Acetaminophen reduced fever only. She c/o burning pain during urination and increased frequency but denies blood in urine.

ROS: positive for dysuria, increased frequency, and lower back pain. Denies hematuria, pyuria, pelvic or perineal pain, vomiting, diarrhea, constipation, numbness and tingling of LE, SOB or headache

PMH: HTN and type 2 DM. Previous hx of recurrent UTI (last episode 1 yr ago). LMP 11 yrs ago; last Pap smear 3 yrs ago; G2P2

Medications: acetaminophen, metformin, and lisinopril. No recent dose changes. NKDA.

FH: not significant

SH: retired teacher, sexually active with husband of 42 yrs

No EtOH, tobacco, or drugs; no recent travel history

Physical Examination

T 38.3 C (101.0 F), BP 129/85 mm Hg, pulse 108/min, respirations 16/min

General: patient appears to be in mild discomfort due to pain

Back: no tenderness on palpation

Abd: no skin abnormalities, +BS × 4Q, no tenderness except in suprapubic/RLQ, and right (R) CVA tenderness

Foot exam: ulcer on plantar surface of left small toe, partially healed

Lower back and neuro: no tenderness on palpation on LS spine, (–) SLR b/l

Data Interpretation

DIAGNOSIS 1. PYELONEPHRITIS

History Findings	Physical Exam Findings
Back pain	Suprapubic tenderness
Fever and chills	Fever, tachycardia
Dysuria	R CVA tenderness
Polyuria	
Fatigue	
Nausea	
h/o recurrent UTIs	

DIAGNOSIS 2. CYSTITIS

History Findings	Physical Exam Findings
Dysuria	Fever
Polyuria	Suprapubic tenderness
Previous UTI	
Diabetes	

DIAGNOSIS 3. NEPHROLITHIASIS

History Findings	Physical Exam Findings
Back pain	Tenderness on palpation, suprapubic & RLQ
Radiation to groin	CVA tenderness
Nausea	Tachycardia
Polyuria	
Dysuria	

Diagnostic Studies

CBC with differential

Urinalysis

Urine culture

CT abdomen/pelvis without IV contrast

Renal U/S

Case Tips and Possible Alternatives

Critical Findings	Case Variations DDX	Important to Communicate
☐ Mid to lower right back pain that radiates to the groin ☐ **Diabetes** ☐ Fever (38.3 C) ☐ Dysuria ☐ Nausea	☐ Appendicitis (atypical presentations in diabetics) ☐ Bladder cancer (30% presents as irritative bladder symptoms)	☐ Importance of glycemic control ☐ Warning signs for diabetic patients ☐ Important control related to long-standing diabetes/HTN
Note: Most patients with diabetes have a fair to good understanding of glycemic control, but physicians should always ascertain the patient's comprehension on daily care, important consultations (ophthalmology, foot care), etc.		

CASE 3: BLOODY STOOLS

Doorway Information

Opening Scenario

Maria Mitchell is a 72-year-old woman who comes to the ER with a history of bloody stool for the past 1 day.

Vital Signs

T 38.3 C (101 F)

BP 108/55 mm Hg

Pulse 105/min

Respirations 16/min

Examinee Tasks

1. Obtain a focused history.

2. Perform a relevant physical exam. Do not perform rectal, pelvic, genitourinary, female breast, or corneal reflex exam.

3. Discuss your initial diagnostic impression and your workup plan with the patient.

4. After leaving the room, complete your Patient Note on the given form.

Communication and Interpersonal Skills Checklist

Fostering the Relationship	Gathering Information	Providing Information
☐ Knocked	☐ Elicited chief complaint	☐ Summarized significant information
☐ Introduced self	☐ Established timeline of patient's CC	☐ Provided diagnostic impression
☐ Clarified role	☐ Used open-ended question	☐ Justified diagnosis with evidence from encounter
☐ Was properly groomed	☐ Used non-leading questions	☐ Assessed patient's need for additional information
☐ Made eye contact	☐ Used closed-ended questions	☐ Encouraged and answered questions
☐ Maintained appropriate distance	☐ Asked one question at a time	☐ Assessed patient's comprehension of probable illness
☐ Displayed confident manner	☐ Did not use medical jargon	
☐ Showed care and concern	☐ Appropriately used "continuers"	
☐ Was respectful and nonjudgmental	☐ Paraphrased	
☐ Established patient's preferred title	☐ Appropriately used transitions	
☐ Used proper draping	☐ Elicited additional concerns	
☐ Focused on patient	☐ Assessed impact on patient's life	
☐ Did not interrupt patient	☐ Checked for patient understanding	
☐ Maintained appropriate and responsive body language		

Making Decisions	Supporting Emotions
☐ Clearly stated next steps in management	☐ Actively listened and validated patient's expectations
☐ **Counseled** patient	☐ Showed empathy and used appropriate reassurances
☐ Agreed to **mutual plan** of action	☐ Inquired about patient's support system
	☐ Managed the **challenge** (here; patient asked, "Will I die?")

History and Physical Examination Checklist

HPI

- ☐ Blood in stool
- ☐ Noticed it yesterday
- ☐ 3 episodes since
  - ☐ Last episode 1 hr ago
  - ☐ Blood mixed with stool
  - ☐ Blood on toilet paper
- ☐ Quantity of blood is "a lot"
- ☐ Lower abd. pain and cramping
- ☐ Feels weak and dizzy when standing up after using the toilet
- ☐ Fever
- ☐ No chills
- ☐ No nausea or vomiting
- ☐ No history of diarrhea
- ☐ No history of constipation
- ☐ No weight loss

PMH

- ☐ No similar episodes in the past
- ☐ HTN
- ☐ Osteoporosis
- ☐ Cholecystectomy at 40
- ☐ Meds: hydrochlorothiazide, multi-vitamins and occasional acetaminophen
- ☐ No anti-inflammatory drugs
- ☐ No anti-coagulants
- ☐ NKDA
- ☐ No past colonoscopy

Family Hx

- ☐ Parent deceased from heart disease in their 80's
- ☐ No family history of colon cancer
- ☐ No family history of IBD

Social Hx

- ☐ No alcohol, no drugs
- ☐ No tobacco use

Physical Examination

- ☐ Washed hands prior to examination
- ☐ Inspected abdomen
- ☐ Healed surgical scar in RUQ
- ☐ Auscultated abdomen in 4 quadrants
- ☐ Percussed abdomen in 4 quadrants
- ☐ Lightly palpated abdomen in 4 quadrants
- ☐ Deeply palpated abdomen in 4 quadrants
- ☐ Checked for guarding and rebound tenderness
- ☐ Auscultated heart (4 areas: A,P,T,M)
- ☐ Examined distal pulses bilaterally

Patient Note

History

CC: 72 yo F c/o bloody stool the past 1 day.

HPI: 3 BMs w/ bright red blood per rectum × 1d w/ lower abd. pain and cramping, no h/o melena a/w BMs in the past, feels "weak and dizzy" when she stands up after going to the bathroom, no previous episodes of rectal bleeding in the past, never had a screening colonoscopy

ROS: positive for hematochezia and fever, denies chills, nausea, vomiting, weight loss, or previous changes in bowel habits

PMH: HTN, osteoporosis

NKDA

Medications: HCTZ, MVI, acetaminophen PRN for pain

PSH: cholecystectomy at age 40

FH: no colon cancer or IBD

SH: no EtOH, tobacco, or drug use

Physical Examination

Vitals: T: 38.3 C, BP: 108/55, P: 105/m, R: 16/m

Gen: Well appearing. NAD

Abd: Well healed surgical scar in RUQ, no other skin lesions; +BS × 4Q, tympanic × 4Q, no palpable masses, soft, NT except in LLQ, and nondistended.

CV: NL S1, S2, regular rhythm, no MRG, peripheral pulses 2+ b/l

---

Data Interpretation

DIAGNOSIS 1. ACUTE DIVERTICULITIS

History Findings	Physical Exam Findings
Hematochezia	No apparent distress (NAD)
Multiple bowel movements	Febrile
Feeling of weakness	No abdominal masses
Dizziness	Tenderness in LLQ
No family history of colon cancer	
Age	

DIAGNOSIS 2. HEMORRHOIDS

History Findings	Physical Exam Findings
Hematochezia	No abdominal masses
Denies any abdominal pain	
No weight loss	
Age	

DIAGNOSIS 3. COLON CANCER

History Findings	Physical Exam Findings
Hematochezia	
No previous colonoscopy	
Age	

Diagnostic Studies

Digital rectal exam

FOBT

CBC w/differential

PT/PTT/INR

CT scan of abd/pelvis

Colonoscopy

Case Tips and Possible Alternatives

Critical Findings	Case Variations DDX	Important to Communicate
☐ **BP: 108/55 mm Hg** ☐ Painless hematochezia ☐ **Positional weakness and dizziness** ☐ No fever, weight loss, vomiting	☐ Angiodysplasia (age >60, tarry stools, anemia) ☐ Colonic polyps ☐ Upper GI bleeding	☐ Importance of screen colonoscopy ☐ Advice about no food/water intake while resolving current situation (possibility of surgery, etc.) ☐ Caution when standing/changing position (fall prevention)
Note: The first step should be to establish the hemodynamic state, as that will dictate how the encounter flows. Check vital signs provided at the door, as that can suggest the seriousness of the case. For CS, emergency cases might merit postponing counseling; however, acknowledge verbally that you are doing that so the patient knows you did not forget.		

CASE 4: CHEST PAIN

Doorway Information

Opening Scenario

Maryann Peters is a 48-year-old woman who presents with chest pain for the past 4 hours.

Vital Signs

T 37 C (98.6 F)

BP 128/58 mm Hg

Pulse 108/min

Respirations 26/min

Oxygen saturation 91% on room air

Examinee Tasks

1. Obtain a focused history.

2. Perform a relevant physical exam. Do not perform rectal, pelvic, genitourinary, female breast, or corneal reflex exam.

3. Discuss your initial diagnostic impression and your workup with the patient.

4. After leaving the room, complete your Patient Note.

Communication and Interpersonal Skills Checklist		
Fostering the Relationship	**Gathering Information**	**Providing Information**
☐ Knocked	☐ Elicited chief complaint	☐ Summarized significant information
☐ Introduced self	☐ Established timeline of patient's CC	☐ Provided diagnostic impression
☐ Clarified role	☐ Used open-ended question	☐ Justified diagnosis with evidence from encounter
☐ Was properly groomed	☐ Used non-leading questions	
☐ Made eye contact	☐ Used closed-ended questions	☐ Assessed patient's need for additional information
☐ Maintained appropriate distance	☐ Asked one question at a time	
☐ Displayed confident manner	☐ Did not use medical jargon	☐ Encouraged and answered questions
☐ Showed care and concern	☐ Appropriately used "continuers"	☐ Assessed patient's comprehension of probable illness
☐ Was respectful and nonjudgmental	☐ Paraphrased	
☐ Established patient's preferred title	☐ Appropriately used transitions	
☐ Used proper draping	☐ Elicited additional concerns	
☐ Focused on patient	☐ Assessed impact on patient's life	
☐ Did not interrupt patient	☐ Checked for patient understanding	
☐ Maintained appropriate and responsive body language		

Making Decisions	Supporting Emotions	
☐ Clearly stated next steps in management	☐ Actively listened and validated patient's expectations	
☐ **Counseled** patient	☐ Showed empathy and used appropriate reassurances	
☐ Agreed to **mutual plan** of action	☐ Inquired about patient's support system	
	☐ Managed the **challenge** (here; patient asked, "Am I having a heart attack?")	

History and Physical Examination Checklist

HPI

- ☐ Chest pain
  - ☐ Substernal
  - ☐ Sharp
  - ☐ Constant
  - ☐ 6/10 intensity
  - ☐ No radiation
- ☐ Duration: 4 hours
- ☐ Breathing makes the pain worse
- ☐ Onset while waiting for her baggage at the airport
- ☐ Recent trip to Japan
- ☐ No diaphoresis
- ☐ No nausea or vomiting
- ☐ SOB: progressively worse
- ☐ Symptoms not improved by rest or ibuprofen
- ☐ No fever or chills
- ☐ No cough or hemoptysis
- ☐ No sick contacts
- ☐ No leg pain or swelling
- ☐ No syncope or palpitations

PMH

- ☐ No similar episodes in the past
- ☐ No GERD
- ☐ HTN
- ☐ Diet controlled–low Na
- ☐ Meds: no prescription, ibuprofen for pain
- ☐ NKDA
- ☐ G1P1
- ☐ No miscarriages
- ☐ + Contraceptive pills

Family Hx:

- ☐ No hx. of blood clots, miscarriages or heart problems

Social Hx

- ☐ Alcohol at social events
- ☐ No recreational drugs
- ☐ Smokes ½ pack/day
  - ☐ 28 years
  - ☐ Trying to quit
- ☐ Married
- ☐ Works as a photographer
- ☐ Is physically active

Physical Examination

- ☐ Washed hands prior to examination
- ☐ Inspection of chest
- ☐ Auscultated heart and carotids
- ☐ Palpated chest for tenderness, location of PMI
  - ☐ Pain not reproduced by palpation
  - ☐ Pain not positional
  - ☐ PMI is not displaced
- ☐ Checked carotids, peripheral pulses and JVP
- ☐ Examined extremities for edema, clubbing, cyanosis, calf tenderness
- ☐ Auscultated lungs
  - ☐ Breathing is painful
- ☐ Assessed chest expansion
- ☐ Assessed tactile fremitus
- ☐ Percussed lungs

Patient Note

History

CC: 48 yo F c/o chest pain for the past 4 hours.

HPI: Substernal pain that is constant, sharp, 6/10 intensity, and non-radiating. Patient thought that lifting heavy luggage upon her arrival from a trip to Japan precipitated the pain. She is experiencing pleuritic chest pain and progressive dyspnea. Resting and ibuprofen provided no relief of pain. No known sick contacts.

ROS: No diaphoresis, nausea, vomiting, palpitations, syncope, fever, chills, cough, hemoptysis. No leg swelling leg pain or general weakness.

PMH: no similar complaints, NKDA, diet-controlled HTN

Meds: Oral contraceptives

FHx: no similar symptoms, no major illnesses, and no history of blood clots

SH: Tobacco 14 pack yrs, trying to quit, ETOH on social events, no illicit drugs

---

Physical Examination

BP 128/58 mm Hg, pulse 108/min, respirations 26/min, T 37 C (98.6 F), and oxygen saturation 91% on room air

General: alert, conscious, and coherent; anxious and uncomfortable; in respiratory distress

CV: Sl and S2 normal; RRR; no m, r, g; PMI not displaced; no carotid bruits; no JVD

Lungs: pain with inspiration and use of accessory muscles; equal chest expansion bilaterally; CTA b/l; no rales, wheezes, rhonchi, or rubs; non-tender on palpation; no dullness on percussion; TVF symmetric and normal b/l.

Extremities: peripheral pulses palpable and equal bilaterally, 2+; no clubbing, cyanosis, or pedal edema

---

Data Interpretation

DIAGNOSIS 1. PULMONARY EMBOLISM

History Findings	Physical Exam Findings
Substernal chest pain, constant, sharp, and non-radiating	Tachypnea
Pleuritic chest pain	Tachycardia
Acute onset of chest pain	
Prolonged travel	Use of accessory muscles
Shortness of breath	Decreased oxygen saturation
Oral contraceptive pills	Clear lungs on auscultation
Tobacco 14 pack yrs	
Female, age	

DIAGNOSIS 2. ACUTE MYOCARDIAL INFARCTION

History Findings	Physical Exam Findings
Substernal chest pain, constant, sharp	Tachypnea
Shortness of breath	Tachycardia
Acute onset of chest pain	Decreased oxygen saturation
Tobacco 14 pack yrs	
History of hypertension	

DIAGNOSIS 3. PNEUMONIA

History Findings	Physical Exam Findings
Substernal chest pain, constant, sharp, and non-radiating	Tachypnea
Pleuritic chest pain	Tachycardia
Shortness of breath	
Tobacco 14 pack yrs	Use of accessory muscles
	Decreased oxygen saturation

Diagnostic Studies

ABG

D-dimer

CBC with diff

EKG, chest x-ray

Troponin/CK-MB

VQ scan or spiral CT

Doppler U/S of lower extremities

Blood culture

BNP

Case Tips and Possible Alternatives

Critical Findings	Case Variations DDX	Important to Communicate
☐ **Acute pleuritic** pain ☐ **Shortness of breath** ☐ Female of reproductive age on oral contraceptives ☐ Smoker ☐ Long distance air travel	☐ Pericarditis (chest pain, worse with inspiration, lying flat, relieved by leaning forward) ☐ GERD ☐ Muscle strain (pinpoint pain on palpation of chest)	☐ Smoking cessation ☐ Risks of smoking and use of oral contraceptives ☐ Air safety tips
Note: Pulmonary embolism is hard to diagnose thus assessing risk factors can provide useful information to guide you.		

CASE 5: IRREGULAR PERIODS

Doorway Information

Opening Scenario

Kathy Hicks is a 23-year-old woman who presents with irregular periods for the past 10 years.

Vital Signs

T 37 C (98.6 F)

BP 120/72 mm Hg

Pulse 84/min

Respirations 12/min

Examinee Tasks

1. Obtain a focused history.

2. Perform a relevant physical exam. Do not perform rectal, pelvic, genitourinary, female breast, or corneal reflex exam.

3. Discuss your initial diagnostic impression and your workup plan with the patient.

4. After leaving the room, complete your Patient Note.

Communication and Interpersonal Skills Checklist

Fostering the Relationship	Gathering Information	Providing Information
☐ Knocked	☐ Elicited chief complaint	☐ Summarized significant information
☐ Introduced self	☐ Established timeline of patient's CC	☐ Provided diagnostic impression
☐ Clarified role	☐ Used open-ended question	☐ Justified diagnosis with evidence from encounter
☐ Was properly groomed	☐ Used non-leading questions	
☐ Made eye contact	☐ Used closed-ended questions	☐ Assessed patient's need for additional information
☐ Maintained appropriate distance	☐ Asked one question at a time	☐ Encouraged and answered questions
☐ Displayed confident manner	☐ Did not use medical jargon	
☐ Showed care and concern	☐ Appropriately used "continuers"	☐ Assessed patient's comprehension of probable illness
☐ Was respectful and nonjudgmental	☐ Paraphrased	
☐ Established patient's preferred title	☐ Appropriately used transitions	
☐ Used proper draping	☐ Elicited additional concerns	
☐ Focused on patient	☐ Assessed impact on patient's life	
☐ Did not interrupt patient	☐ Checked for patient understanding	
☐ Maintained appropriate and responsive body language		

Making Decisions	Supporting Emotions
☐ Clearly stated next steps in management	☐ Actively listened and validated patient's expectations
☐ **Counseled** patient	☐ Showed empathy and used appropriate reassurances
☐ Agreed to **mutual plan** of action	☐ Inquired about patient's support system
	☐ Managed the **challenge** (here; patient asked, "Will I have problems getting pregnant?")

History and Physical Examination Checklist

HPI

- ☐ Irregular menstrual periods
- ☐ Duration: 10 years
- ☐ First period at 13
- ☐ Periods were never regular
  - ☐ Every 2-3 mos
- ☐ Gained 15 lbs in last 5 years
  - ☐ Consistent with poor diet
- ☐ No breast tenderness
- ☐ No nipple discharge
- ☐ LMP 8 weeks ago
- ☐ Trying to get pregnant
- ☐ Hirsutism
- ☐ No increased urinary frequency
- ☐ No excessive thirst
- ☐ No cold/heat intolerance
- ☐ No skin, hair, or nail changes
- ☐ No constipation

PMH

- ☐ History of menstrual cramps
- ☐ Takes ibuprofen for menstrual cramps
- ☐ Meds: topical benzoyl peroxide for acne, folic acid and multivitamin supplement.
- ☐ Acne since puberty
- ☐ NKDA
- ☐ G0P0
- ☐ No STDs

Family Hx

- ☐ Mother 58 yo has diabetes
- ☐ Sister 26 yo had diabetes while pregnant

Social Hx

- ☐ No alcohol
- ☐ No recreational drugs
- ☐ No tobacco use
- ☐ Married
- ☐ Monogamous

Physical Examination

- ☐ Washed hands prior to examination
- ☐ Inspected skin: facial acne and hirsutism noted
- ☐ Inspected abdomen: obese abdomen
- ☐ Auscultated 4 quadrants of abdomen
- ☐ Percussed 4 quadrants of abdomen
- ☐ Palpated 4 quadrants of abdomen
  - ☐ Light palpation
  - ☐ Deep palpation if no tenderness upon light palpation
- ☐ Palpated thyroid

Patient Note

History

CC: 23 yo F c/o irregular periods for the past 10 years.

HPI: cycles every 2-3 mos, menstrual periods irregular since menarche at age 13, + hirsutism, + dysmenorrhea, + facial acne, unintentional weight gain of 15 pounds/5 yrs, no changes in hair or nails, no cold intolerance, no constipation

ROS: - for seborrhea, hyperhidrosis, hidradenitis suppurativa, temporal hair balding, increased muscle bulk and voice deepening; no h/o breast tenderness, lactation, polydipsia, polyphagia or change in urinary habits or frequency

NKDA

Meds: benzoyl peroxide (topical), folic acid, multivitamin supplement, ibuprofen (for dysmenorrhea)

No hospitalizations, surgeries, or trauma

FH: father and brother are alive and healthy, mother alive and diabetic, sister with gestational diabetes

OB/Gyn: LMP 8 wks ago; G0 P0

SH: No EtOH/ tobacco/ illicit drugs; diet: processed foods, high in carbohydrate and fat, monogamous with husband, No STDs

Physical Examination

T 98.6 F, BP 120/72 mm Hg, pulse 84/min, respirations 12/min

General: alert, conscious, and coherent; not in acute distress

HEENT: facial acne and hirsutism noted; no thyromegaly

Abd: obese; no abdominal striae; BS × 4Q, tympanic × 4Q; soft, non-tender, non-distended; no organomegaly

Data Interpretation

Diagnosis 1. Polycystic Ovarian Syndrome

History Findings	Physical Exam Findings
Irregular periods for 10 yrs	Facial acne
History of acne	Hirsutism
Dysmenorrhea	Abd obese
Unintentional weight gain of 15 pounds in 5 yrs	
G0P0	
FH of DM	

DIAGNOSIS 2. HYPOTHYROIDISM

History Findings	Physical Exam Findings
Irregular periods for 10 yrs	Abdominal obesity
Unintentional weight gain of 15 pounds in 5 yrs	

DIAGNOSIS 3. CUSHING SYNDROME

History Findings	Physical Exam Findings
Irregular periods for 10 yrs	Abdominal obesity
Unintentional weight gain of 15 pounds in 5 yrs	Facial acne
	Hirsutism

Diagnostic Studies

Pelvic exam

Serum hCG

Pelvic/transvaginal U/S

OGTT, serum insulin level

Total cholesterol, HDL, LDL, TG

TSH, LH, FSH

24-hour urinary cortisol excretion

Total testosterone, androgen levels

Case Tips and Possible Alternatives

Critical Findings	Case Variations DDX	Important to Communicate
☐ **Irregular menstrual periods** ☐ **Hirsutism** ☐ Dysmenorrhea ☐ Facial acne ☐ Unintentional weight gain ☐ **No** heat/cold intolerance	☐ Ovarian hyperthecosis (usually seen in older, post-menopausal women) ☐ Ovarian cancer (BRCA1/2, family history, etc.)	☐ Lifestyle change (diet and exercise + importance of risk due to diabetes in family history) ☐ Family planning and reproductive health
Note: When possible, ask patients of reproductive age about their future goals and expectations for pregnancy.		

CASE 6: SORE THROAT

Doorway Information

Opening Scenario

Alex Pallon is a 16-year-old male who presents with sore throat for the past 1 day.

Vital Signs

T 38.3 C (101.0 F)

BP 122/60 mm Hg

Pulse 98/min

Respirations 12/min

Oxygen saturation 98% on room air

Examinee Tasks

1. Obtain a focused history.

2. Perform a relevant physical exam. Do not perform rectal, pelvic, genitourinary, female breast, or corneal reflex exam.

3. Discuss your initial diagnostic impression and your workup plan with the patient and his parent.

4. After leaving the room, complete your Patient Note.

Communication and Interpersonal Skills Checklist

Fostering the Relationship	Gathering Information	Providing Information
☐ Knocked	☐ Elicited chief complaint	☐ Summarized significant information
☐ Introduced self	☐ Established timeline of patient's CC	☐ Provided diagnostic impression
☐ Clarified role	☐ Used open-ended question	☐ Justified diagnosis with evidence from encounter
☐ Was properly groomed	☐ Used non-leading questions	☐ Assessed patient's need for additional information
☐ Made eye contact	☐ Used closed-ended questions	
☐ Maintained appropriate distance	☐ Asked one question at a time	☐ Encouraged and answered questions
☐ Displayed confident manner	☐ Did not use medical jargon	☐ Assessed patient's comprehension of probable illness
☐ Showed care and concern	☐ Appropriately used "continuers"	
☐ Was respectful and nonjudgmental	☐ Paraphrased	
☐ Established patient's preferred title	☐ Appropriately used transitions	
☐ Used proper draping	☐ Elicited additional concerns	
☐ Focused on patient	☐ Assessed impact on patient's life	
☐ Did not interrupt patient	☐ Checked for patient understanding	
☐ Maintained appropriate and responsive body language		

Making Decisions	Supporting Emotions
☐ Clearly stated next steps in management	☐ Actively listened and validated patient's expectations
☐ **Counseled** patient	☐ Showed empathy and used appropriate reassurances
☐ Agreed to **mutual plan** of action	☐ Inquired about patient's support system
	☐ Managed the **challenge** (here; patient asked, "Can you give me a prescription for antibiotics?")

History and Physical Examination Checklist

HPI

- ☐ Sore throat
- ☐ Sharp pain
  - ☐ Started 1 day ago
  - ☐ Progressively worse
  - ☐ 8/10 intensity
  - ☐ Greater on the right side
  - ☐ Increased with swallowing
  - ☐ No radiation
- ☐ Symptoms have not improved with rest or ibuprofen
- ☐ Fever (101°F in the morning)
- ☐ Fatigue (left soccer practice early)
- ☐ Chills
- ☐ Dull headache
- ☐ Nasal discharge
- ☐ No cough or respiratory distress
- ☐ No rashes
- ☐ No abdominal pain, anorexia, or weight loss
- ☐ No nausea or vomiting
- ☐ Sick contacts (soccer teammates)

PMH

- ☐ No similar episodes in the past
- ☐ Meds: no prescription meds, + ibuprofen
- ☐ NKDA

Family Hx:

- ☐ 9 mo-old brother w/recent cold

Social Hx

- ☐ No alcohol
- ☐ No recreational drugs
- ☐ Smoked 4 cigarettes over the past 6 mos
- ☐ Not sexually active
- ☐ Physically active (plays soccer)

Physical Examination

- ☐ Washed hands prior to examination
- ☐ Inspected skin for rashes
- ☐ Inspected both nares
- ☐ Inspected, palpated ears bilaterally
- ☐ Performed bilateral otoscopic exam
- ☐ Examined mouth, posterior pharynx and elevation of palate
- ☐ Palpated sinuses for tenderness
- ☐ Palpated posterior auricular lymph nodes
- ☐ Palpated anterior cervical lymph nodes
- ☐ Palpated posterior cervical lymph nodes
- ☐ Palpated submandibular lymph nodes
- ☐ Palpated submental lymph nodes
- ☐ Auscultated both lung fields
- ☐ Percussed thorax

Patient Note

History

CC: 16 yo M c/o sore throat for 1 day.

HPI: 8/10 intensity. He felt tired yesterday and left soccer practice early. A few teammates have also been ill. He states the right throat area hurts more than the left, and the pain is mostly a sharp pain, not radiating anywhere. Pain aggravated by swallowing and alleviated by nothing.

ROS: Fever, chills, nasal discharge, fatigue, and dull headache. Denies abdominal pain, nausea, vomiting, anorexia, weight loss, rashes, respiratory distress, cough.

PMH: no previous episodes. NKDA

Meds: no Rx meds, OTC ibuprofen

Hosp/illness/trauma: none

Family Hx: 9 month old brother had a cold recently.

Social History: smoked 4 cigarettes over the last 6 mos. No EtOH or drugs. Lives at home with mother, father, and brother. Pt is not sexually active. He plays soccer.

Physical Exam

T 101.0 F, BP 122/60, pulse 98, respirations 12, oxygen saturation 98% on room air

General: patient appears uncomfortable but not in acute distress.

HEENT: Ears (TM visualized, no bulging or erythema, no tenderness elicited). Scant clear discharge from nares B/L. Throat - erythema noted in posterior pharynx, no exudates noted, and tonsils not enlarged. Sinus - no tenderness on palpation. Neck - no LAD

Lungs: CTA b/l, no wheezes/crepitations/rales/rhonchi

Skin: no erythema or rash noted

Data Interpretation

DIAGNOSIS 1. VIRAL PHARYNGITIS

History Findings	Physical Exam Findings
Sore throat	Erythema on posterior pharynx
Odynophagia	Fever
Fatigue	No lymphadenopathy
Sick contacts	No exudates
Nasal discharge	
Sudden onset	

DIAGNOSIS 2. STREP PHARYNGITIS

History Findings	Physical Exam Findings
Sore throat	Erythema on posterior pharynx
Odynophagia	Fever
Fatigue	
Sick contacts	
Headache	

DIAGNOSIS 3. INFECTIOUS MONONUCLEOSIS

History Findings	Physical Exam Findings
Sore throat	Erythema on posterior pharynx
Odynophagia	Fever
Fatigue	No nasal discharge
Sick contacts	
Age (primarily young adults)	

Diagnostic Studies

CBC with differential, with peripheral blood smear

Rapid strep test

Throat culture

Monospot test

Case Tips and Possible Alternatives

Critical Findings	Case Variations DDX	Important to Communicate
☐ Age ☐ Sore throat ☐ **Temp: 38.3 C (101 F)** ☐ Odynophagia ☐ Fatigue ☐ Sick contacts	☐ Peritonsillar abscess (high fever, in great distress) ☐ Mumps (one-sided neck pain, pain worse when consuming acidic foods)	☐ Alarming signs and symptoms that may require immediate medical attention ☐ Increased rest, consumption of fluids ☐ Washing of hands and ways to decrease spread
Note: When facing an underage patient, it is imperative to understand who can (and needs to) consent.		

CASE 7: HEARING LOSS

Doorway Information

Opening Scenario

Ron Ryder is a 53-year-old man who comes to the office today because of hearing loss for the past 5 years.

Vital Signs

T 37 C (98.6 F)

BP 128/72 mm Hg

Pulse 80/min

Respirations 12/min

Examinee Tasks

1. Obtain a focused history.

2. Perform a relevant physical exam. Do not perform rectal, pelvic, genitourinary, or corneal reflex exam.

3. Discuss your initial diagnostic impression and your workup plan with the patient.

4. After leaving the room, complete your Patient Note on the given form.

Communication and Interpersonal Skills Checklist

Fostering the Relationship	Gathering Information	Providing Information
☐ Knocked	☐ Elicited chief complaint	☐ Summarized significant information
☐ Introduced self	☐ Established timeline of patient's CC	☐ Provided diagnostic impression
☐ Clarified role	☐ Used open-ended question	☐ Justified diagnosis with evidence from encounter
☐ Was properly groomed	☐ Used non-leading questions	☐ Assessed patient's need for additional information
☐ Made eye contact	☐ Used closed-ended questions	☐ Encouraged and answered questions
☐ Maintained appropriate distance	☐ Asked one question at a time	☐ Assessed patient's comprehension of probable illness
☐ Displayed confident manner	☐ Did not use medical jargon	
☐ Showed care and concern	☐ Appropriately used "continuers"	
☐ Was respectful and nonjudgmental	☐ Paraphrased	
☐ Established patient's preferred title	☐ Appropriately used transitions	
☐ Used proper draping	☐ Elicited additional concerns	
☐ Focused on patient	☐ Assessed impact on patient's life	
☐ Did not interrupt patient	☐ Checked for patient understanding	
☐ Maintained appropriate and responsive body language		

Making Decisions	Supporting Emotions
☐ Clearly stated next steps in management	☐ Actively listened and validated patient's expectations
☐ **Counseled** patient	☐ Showed empathy and used appropriate reassurances
☐ Agreed to **mutual plan** of action	☐ Inquired about patient's support system
	☐ Managed the **challenge** (here; patient has difficulty hearing your questions)

History and Physical Examination Checklist

HPI

- ☐ Hearing loss
  - ☐ Bilateral
  - ☐ Noticed 5 years ago
  - ☐ Progressed slowly over the years
  - ☐ Initially a problem with large crowds that have lots of background noise
  - ☐ Lately, can't hear his wife at dinner table
- ☐ No history of ear infections
- ☐ No trauma
- ☐ Uses Q tips to clean wax
  - ☐ No pain
  - ☐ No blood
  - ☐ Minimal wax
- ☐ Tried OTC drops to remove wax
  - ☐ Did not improve hearing
  - ☐ Ears seemed clean of wax
- ☐ Headache
- ☐ No discharge from ear
- ☐ No fever
- ☐ No numbness
- ☐ No tingling
- ☐ No weakness
- ☐ No dizziness
- ☐ No spinning of the room or unsteadiness
- ☐ No ringing in the ears

PMH

- ☐ No previous hospitalizations or surgeries
- ☐ Meds: no Rx meds. Uses aspirin PRN for headaches (provides modest relief)
- ☐ NKDA
- ☐ Never used hearing aids

Family Hx

- ☐ No family history of hearing loss

Social Hx

- ☐ He is a farmer
- ☐ Drives loud tractor
- ☐ Listens to rock music with headphones
- ☐ Alcohol: socially (2 beers/week × 20 years)
- ☐ No recreational drugs
- ☐ No tobacco use
- ☐ Married, sexually active w/wife only; regular condom use
- ☐ 3 small children
- ☐ Sx are affecting his quality of life

Physical Examination

- ☐ Washed hands prior to examination
- ☐ Tested auditory acuity b/l (finger rub or whispered voice)
  - ☐ Cannot hear finger rub bilaterally
- ☐ Inspected external ears
- ☐ Performed otoscopic exam bilaterally
- ☐ Performed Rinne test and compare AC with BC b/l
  - ☐ Bone conduction is greater than air conduction
- ☐ Performed Weber test and observe for lateralization to any side
  - ☐ Does not localize to either side
- ☐ Performed posterior auricular, anterior cervical, and posterior cervical lymph node exam
- ☐ Observed gait
- ☐ Performed Romberg test
- ☐ CN and nystagmus

Patient Note

History

CC: 53 yo M c/o hearing loss × 5 years

HPI: B/l, insidious, progressively worsening, initially had trouble hearing in loud social environment but now has trouble hearing his wife at the dinner table, no diurnal variation, + headphones use and constant exposure to loud noises d/t tractor driving, denies trauma to head, ears or previous falls, cleans ears w/ Q-tips, current symptoms are impacting to his quality of life, never used hearing aids in the past

ROS: + occasional headaches, + paradoxical hypersensitivity to loud sounds, no fever, no ear pain, no numbness, tingling, or weakness in any part of the face or body, no loss of equilibrium, no tinnitus, no vertigo, no d/c or blood from ears, no rhinorrhea

PMH: no other major illness NKDA

Meds: no Rx meds, + aspirin PRN for headaches (provides modest relief) No h/o hospitalizations or surgeries

FHx: no similar CC; no other major illness

SHx: farmer; 2 beers / wk × 20 yrs; no h/o smoking or recreational drug use, sexually active with wife only, uses condoms regularly

---

Physical Examination

T 37 C (98.6 F), BP: 128/72 mm Hg, pulse: 80/min, respirations: 12/min

General: pleasant but cannot hear well despite speaking loudly

HEENT: NL outer ear, TM seen, no evidence of hemotympanum, otorrhea, exudates or erythema, no polyps, minimal ear wax impaction, Weber's test: no lateralization, Rinne's test: AC > BC b/l, no LAD; negative Battle sign.

NEURO: NL gait, Romberg negative, symmetric hearing loss detected b/l, other CNs intact.

Data Interpretation

Diagnosis 1. Presbycusis

History Findings	Physical Exam Findings
B/l high frequency hearing loss that started 5 yrs ago	Symmetric hearing loss (b/l)
Progressively worsened	Ear inspection: no erythema, polyps, or exudates; minimal ear wax
Farmer, exposure to loud noises	
Insidious hearing loss from high to low pitch	
Age	
No fever	
No pain	
No numbness or tingling or vertigo	

Diagnosis 2. Ruptured Tympanic Membrane

History Findings	Physical Exam Findings
Hearing loss	hearing loss
No fever	Ear inspection: no erythema, polyps, or exudates; minimal ear wax
No pain	
Cleans ears with Q-tips	
No numbness or tingling	
No vertigo	

Diagnosis 3. Aspirin Toxicity

History Findings	Physical Exam Findings
Bilateral hearing loss	Bilateral hearing loss
Hx of aspirin use	Ear inspection: no erythema, polyps, or exudates; minimal ear wax

Diagnostic Studies

CBC w/ differential

Serum salicylate acid level

Audiogram

Case Tips and Possible Alternatives

Critical Findings	Case Variations DDX	Important to Communicate
☐ **Bilateral** hearing loss ☐ Age ☐ Progressive ☐ Has been a farmer for many years	☐ Acoustic neuroma (one-sided hearing loss, tinnitus, vertigo, headache) ☐ Cholesteatoma (conductive hearing loss, drainage and granulation tissue in the ear canal, dizziness)	☐ Avoiding constant loud sounds ☐ Hearing protection (earplugs, earmuffs) ☐ Check medication list for hearing risks
Note: Environmental hearing loss is common, thus it is useful to know people's job type, duration, and environment which might put them at risk for hearing loss.		

CASE 8: "SOMETHING IS WRONG WITH MY DAD."

Doorway Information

Opening Scenario

Debby Longo is on the telephone. She is the daughter of Edward Bello, who is 75-years-old. She tells you "Something is wrong with my father" after visiting him at his home earlier today.

Vital Signs

Not available

Examinee Tasks

1. Obtain a focused history.

2. You will not be required to perform a physical exam in this case.

3. Discuss your initial diagnostic impression and your workup plan with the patient's daughter.

4. After leaving the room, complete your Patient Note. Leave the physical exam portion blank.

Communication and Interpersonal Skills Checklist

Fostering the Relationship	Gathering Information	Providing Information
☐ Introduced self ☐ Clarified role ☐ Displayed confident manner ☐ Showed care and concern ☐ Was respectful and nonjudgmental ☐ Established preferred title ☐ Did not interrupt	☐ Elicited chief complaint ☐ Established timeline of patient's CC ☐ Used open-ended question ☐ Used non-leading questions ☐ Used closed-ended questions ☐ Asked one question at a time ☐ Did not use medical jargon ☐ Appropriately used "continuers" ☐ Paraphrased ☐ Appropriately used transitions ☐ Elicited additional concerns ☐ Assessed impact on patient's life ☐ Checked for understanding	☐ Summarized significant information ☐ Provided diagnostic impression ☐ Justified diagnosis with evidence from encounter ☐ Assessed need for additional information ☐ Encouraged and answered questions ☐ Assessed comprehension of probable illness

Making Decisions	Supporting Emotions
☐ Clearly stated next steps in management ☐ **Counseled** relative ☐ Agreed to **mutual plan** of action	☐ Actively listened and validated expectations ☐ Showed empathy and used appropriate reassurances ☐ Inquired about patient's support system ☐ Managed the **challenge** (here; daughter worried for patient)

History and Physical Examination Checklist

HPI

- ☐ Slurred speech
- ☐ Sudden onset
- ☐ Started during breakfast
- ☐ Single episode
- ☐ Duration: 20 mins
- ☐ Difficulty picking up a jar of jelly
- ☐ Unable to hold a cup of coffee
- ☐ Patient stumbled when he tried to stand
- ☐ Difficulty moving right leg
- ☐ + headache
- ☐ No dysphagia or dystonia
- ☐ No loss of consciousness
- ☐ No bowel or bladder incontinence
- ☐ No visual problems, tinnitus or hearing loss
- ☐ No loss of sensation
- ☐ No jerky movements of limbs
- ☐ No fever
- ☐ No confusion
- ☐ Drooping face

PMH

- ☐ High cholesterol
- ☐ Last test 6 mos ago 110 mg/dl LDL
- ☐ No HTN
- ☐ No diabetes
- ☐ No heart disease
- ☐ No history of stroke
- ☐ No previous surgery or hospitalization
- ☐ NKDA
- ☐ Meds: aspirin and atorvastatin

Family Hx

- ☐ Father died of stroke at age 92

Social Hx

- ☐ Retired malpractice lawyer
- ☐ No smoking
- ☐ Alcohol 1-2 times per month
- ☐ No recreational drugs
- ☐ Plays golf on weekends

Physical Examination

No physical exam

Patient Note

History

CC: 75 yo M whose daughter c/o "Something is wrong with my father."

HPI: Hx provided by daughter on phone. 75 y/o man c/o slurred speech for 20 min. Sudden onset yesterday morning. No clear precipitating factor. Had trouble picking up jar of jelly with R hand. He stumbled getting out of chair due to difficulty moving his R leg but did not fall. His symptoms resolved spontaneously. He also reported a headache. No difficulty swallowing. His wife noticed his face looked "little different" during the episode. No further episodes.

ROS: (+)Headache. (−) h/o fever, confusion, LOC, vision changes, tinnitus, hearing loss, loss of sensation, bowel/bladder incontinence, dysphagia, dystonia, tonic-clonic movements.

PMH: h/o hyperlipidemia; no h/o similar episodes in past; last physical 6 mos ago–lipid panel normal.

Meds: Aspirin daily, atorvastatin compliant; NKDA ; no h/o hosp or surgeries; sleep not disturbed

Family Hx: no similar CC; father died of a stroke at age 92

Social Hx: he drinks 1-2 drinks/month; no h/o smoking or rec drugs

Physical Exam

N/A

Data Interpretation

Diagnosis 1. Transient Ischemic Attack

History Findings	Physical Exam Findings
Sudden onset of slurring speech	
Duration 20 min	
R hand weakness	
Transient R leg weakness	
Face looked "little different"	
No h/o fever, confusion, LOC, incontinence, tonic-clonic movements	
Age	
Elevated cholesterol	

DIAGNOSIS 2. CEREBROVASCULAR ACCIDENT

History Findings	Physical Exam Findings
Sudden onset of slurred speech	
R hand weakness	
Transient R leg weakness	
Face looked "little different"	
Negative h/o fever, tonic-clonic movements	
Elevated cholesterol	

Diagnostic Studies

Physical examination

Cholesterol, HDL, LDL, triglycerides, CBC, electrolytes, glucose, PT, PTT

EKG

Carotid U/S

CT scan of head without contrast

MRI/MRA of brain

Case Tips and Possible Alternatives

Must not Miss	Case Variations DDX	Important to Communicate
☐ **Headache** ☐ Slurred speech ☐ Episode duration: **20 min** ☐ Resolved spontaneously ☐ R UE & LE weakness ☐ No LOC	☐ Carotid artery dissection (headache and face pain, *amaurosis fugax*, pulsatile tinnitus) ☐ Subarachnoid hemorrhage (sudden severe headache, nausea, focal neuro deficits, LOC, seizures)	☐ Diet and monitoring of hyperlipidemia ☐ Stroke warnings (signs and symptoms) ☐ Safety, fall prevention, activity, meds ☐ Emergency plan
Note: For patients presenting with neurological problems, pay attention to timing and duration of signs and symptoms, as well as unnoticed deficits particular to the patient. Sometimes deficits are subtle and might go unnoticed, especially in elderly patients.		

CASE 9: SEVERE HEADACHE

Doorway Information

Opening Scenario

Patrick Davis is a 45-year-old man who comes to the ER because of a severe headache for the past 4 hours.

Vital Signs

T 37.8 C (100 F)

BP 169/108 mm Hg

Pulse 48/min

Respirations 12/min

Examinee Tasks

1. Obtain a focused history.

2. Perform a relevant physical exam. Do not perform rectal, pelvic, genitourinary, or corneal reflex exam.

3. Discuss your initial diagnostic impression and your workup plan with the patient.

4. After leaving the room, complete the Patient Note.

Communication and Interpersonal Skills Checklist		
Fostering the Relationship	**Gathering Information**	**Providing Information**
☐ Knocked ☐ Introduced self ☐ Clarified role ☐ Was properly groomed ☐ Made eye contact ☐ Maintained appropriate distance ☐ Displayed confident manner ☐ Showed care and concern ☐ Was respectful and nonjudgmental ☐ Established patient's preferred title ☐ Used proper draping ☐ Focused on patient ☐ Did not interrupt patient ☐ Maintained appropriate and responsive body language	☐ Elicited chief complaint ☐ Established timeline of patient's CC ☐ Used open-ended question ☐ Used non-leading questions ☐ Used closed-ended questions ☐ Asked one question at a time ☐ Did not use medical jargon ☐ Appropriately used "continuers" ☐ Paraphrased ☐ Appropriately used transitions ☐ Elicited additional concerns ☐ Assessed impact on patient's life ☐ Checked for patient understanding	☐ Summarized significant information ☐ Provided diagnostic impression ☐ Justified diagnosis with evidence from encounter ☐ Assessed patient's need for additional information ☐ Encouraged and answered questions ☐ Assessed patient's comprehension of probable illness

Making Decisions	**Supporting Emotions**
☐ Clearly stated next steps in management ☐ **Counseled** patient ☐ Agreed to **mutual plan** of action	☐ Actively listened and validated patient's expectations ☐ Showed empathy and used appropriate reassurances ☐ Inquired about patient's support system ☐ Managed the **challenge** (here; patient asked, "Can you make it stop?")

History and Physical Examination Checklist

HPI

- ☐ Headache
  - ☐ 10/10 intensity
  - ☐ Persistent
  - ☐ Radiation to neck and back
  - ☐ Started while coaching his daughter's Little League game
- ☐ Duration: 4 hours
- ☐ Worse with cough
- ☐ Worse with movement of head
- ☐ Nausea
- ☐ No vomiting
- ☐ No LOC
- ☐ No trauma
- ☐ No seizures
- ☐ No fever
- ☐ No chills
- ☐ No photophobia
- ☐ No confusion
- ☐ No changes in vision
- ☐ No recent illness
- ☐ No sick contacts
- ☐ No vertigo or tinnitus

PMH

- ☐ No similar episodes in the past
- ☐ No hospitalizations or surgeries
- ☐ Meds: 400 mg of ibuprofen earlier
- ☐ NKDA

Family Hx

- ☐ No family history of stroke, vascular disease, or heart disease
- ☐ Maternal uncle has polycystic kidney disease on hemodialysis

Social Hx

- ☐ Alcohol: 1-2 beers 5 days a week × 10 years
- ☐ Snorts cocaine on most weekends
- ☐ No IV drug use
- ☐ Smokes
  - ☐ 1-2 pack/day
  - ☐ 10 years
- ☐ Married, sexually active with wife only
- ☐ Works as a bartender at a local bar

Physical Examination

- ☐ Washed hands prior to examination
- ☐ Performed mental status exam
- ☐ Performed inspection of head
- ☐ Performed palpation of head
- ☐ Performed fundoscopic exam
- ☐ Examined CNII–XII
- ☐ Assessed motor strength bilaterally
- ☐ Examined DTRs
- ☐ Checked sensation with at least 2 modalities (light, sharp/dull, proprioception)
- ☐ Assessed cerebellar function (dysmetria, dysdiadochokinesia, or Romberg)
- ☐ Examined for Babinski reflex
  - ☐ Negative Babinski
- ☐ Tested for nuchal rigidity and performed Brudzinski or Kernig test
  - ☐ + Nuchal rigidity
  - ☐ + Brudzinski

Patient Note

History

CC: 45 yo M c/o severe headache for the past 4 hours.

HPI: He reports having a generalized headache. The headache is sharp with intensity of 10/10, radiates down his neck and spine, is aggravated by movement, and is associated with nausea. He has no relief with OTC analgesics. He describes it as the "worst headache of my life." He denies sick contact, recent URI. He admits to using cocaine on most weekends, but denies other drug use.

ROS: + nausea. Denies vomiting, fever, chills, seizures, confusion, photophobia, vertigo, trauma, tinnitus, and LOC.

PMH/PSHx: No h/o similar symptoms in the past, no other major illness, No h/o hospitalizations or surgeries.

NKDA

Meds: ibuprofen OTC for relief; no regular meds or supplements

Family Hx: No similar CC; uncle on dialysis for PCKD

Social Hx: 1-2 beers 5 days/wk × 10 yrs; 1-2 packs of cigs/day × 10 yrs; h/o cocaine snorting - no IVDU, sexually active with wife only; uses condoms regularly

Physical Examination

BP 169/108 mm Hg, pulse 48/min, T 37.8 C (100 F), respirations 12/min

GA: Appears confused and in moderate distress

A&O × 2: to person and place

Eyes: no papilledema or optic disc blurring on fundoscopy

CN II–XII intact

LE: motor: 5/5 b/I DTR: 2+ throughout

Sensory: light, sharp/dull & proprioception intact b/I

No dysmetria, dysdiadochokinesia

+Nuchal rigidity, +Brudzinski, –Babinski

Data Interpretation

DIAGNOSIS 1. RUPTURED CEREBRAL ANEURYSM

History Findings	Physical Exam Findings
Sudden, severe generalized headache	Hypertensive, afebrile
intensity of 10/10 "worst headache of life"	A&O × 2: can't remember date
Aggravated by movement and no relief with analgesics	Brudzinski test: positive
Associated with nausea	+ Nuchal rigidity
Pain radiating down neck and spine	
No hx of fevers, chills, sick contact, trauma	
Family h/o PCKD	
Smoker	

DIAGNOSIS 2. SPONTANEOUS INTRACEREBRAL HEMORRHAGE

History Findings	Physical Exam Findings
Generalized headache	Hypertensive
Sharp headache, intensity 10/10	A&O × 2 : can't remember date
Aggravated by movement and no relief with OTC pain meds	Brudzinski test: positive
Assoc with nausea	+ Nuchal rigidity
Negative h/o trauma	
h/o cocaine-snorting	

DIAGNOSIS 3. MENINGITIS

History Findings	Physical Exam Findings
Generalized headache	Hypertensive, bradycardia
Severe headache	A&O × 2 : can't remember date
Aggravated by movement and no relief with OTC pain meds	No papilledema or optic disc blurring on fundoscopy
Assoc with nausea	Brudzinski test: positive
	+ Nuchal rigidity

Diagnostic Studies

CBC w diff

Urine toxicology

CT head without contrast

Lumbar puncture

MRI brain, MRA brain

Case Tips and Possible Alternatives

Critical Findings	Case Variations DDX	Important to Communicate
☐ 10/10 headache ☐ Nausea ☐ Not relieved by analgesics ☐ No LOC ☐ Cocaine use (snorting)	☐ Acute subdural hematoma (4–21 days- Hx of trauma, usually age >40) ☐ Cluster headache (intense unilateral headache, ptosis, ipsilateral lacrimation, nasal stuffiness)	☐ Probable emergency case: advice about not eating/drinking in case of imminent surgical intervention ☐ Importance of BP control ☐ Facilitating and educating about effects of Cocaine use
Note: When facing patients with drug use/abuse, provide a safe space and non-judgmental attitude, which will invite honest answers. When time allows, ask what the patient finds beneficial about their drug consumption; this might reveal underlying issues (sometimes drugs or alcohol can be a form of unintentional self-medication).		

CASE 10: SEVERE ABDOMINAL PAIN

Doorway Information

Opening Scenario

Michelle Thompson is a 31-year-old woman who comes to the ER because of severe abdominal pain for the past 5 hours.

Vital Signs

T 38.3 C (101.0 F)

BP 102/60 mm Hg

Pulse 109/min

Respirations 27/min

Examinee Tasks

1. Obtain a focused history.

2. Perform a relevant physical exam. Do not perform rectal, pelvic, genitourinary, female breast, or corneal reflex exam.

3. Discuss your initial diagnostic impression and your workup plan with the patient.

4. After leaving the room, complete your Patient Note.

Communication and Interpersonal Skills Checklist

Fostering the Relationship	Gathering Information	Providing Information
☐ Knocked	☐ Elicited chief complaint	☐ Summarized significant information
☐ Introduced self	☐ Established timeline of patient's CC	☐ Provided diagnostic impression
☐ Clarified role	☐ Used open-ended question	☐ Justified diagnosis with evidence from encounter
☐ Was properly groomed	☐ Used non-leading questions	☐ Assessed patient's need for additional information
☐ Made eye contact	☐ Used closed-ended questions	☐ Encouraged and answered questions
☐ Maintained appropriate distance	☐ Asked one question at a time	☐ Assessed patient's comprehension of probable illness
☐ Displayed confident manner	☐ Did not use medical jargon	
☐ Showed care and concern	☐ Appropriately used "continuers"	
☐ Was respectful and nonjudgmental	☐ Paraphrased	
☐ Established patient's preferred title	☐ Appropriately used transitions	
☐ Used proper draping	☐ Elicited additional concerns	
☐ Focused on patient	☐ Assessed impact on patient's life	
☐ Did not interrupt patient	☐ Checked for patient understanding	
☐ Maintained appropriate and responsive body language		

Making Decisions	Supporting Emotions
☐ Clearly stated next steps in management	☐ Actively listened and validated patient's expectations
☐ **Counseled** patient	☐ Showed empathy and used appropriate reassurances
☐ Agreed to **mutual plan** of action	☐ Inquired about patient's support system
	☐ Managed the **challenge** (here; patient asked, "Will I need surgery?")

History and Physical Examination Checklist

HPI

- [ ] Abdominal pain
    - [ ] LUQ and RUQ
    - [ ] Dull
    - [ ] 10/10 intensity
    - [ ] Constant
    - [ ] Sudden onset
    - [ ] Radiates to the back
    - [ ] Not related to food intake
- [ ] Duration: 5 hours
- [ ] Aspirin did not alleviate her symptoms
- [ ] Leaning forward alleviates pain
- [ ] Laying supine exacerbates pain
- [ ] No fever
- [ ] No chills
- [ ] No diarrhea
- [ ] No cough
- [ ] No dyspnea
- [ ] No chest pain
- [ ] No dark stools
- [ ] No sick contacts
- [ ] 3 episodes of emesis today
    - [ ] Non-bloody
    - [ ] Non-bilious
    - [ ] Persistent nausea for several hours

PMH

- [ ] 1 similar episode in the past
    - [ ] 2 years ago
    - [ ] Admitted to the intensive care unit
    - [ ] Does not recall her diagnosis or treatment
- [ ] Recurrent urinary tract infections
- [ ] No h/o DM
- [ ] No surgeries
- [ ] Meds: no prescription meds; uses ASA regularly
- [ ] NKDA
- [ ] No children
- [ ] LMP 10 days ago

Family Hx

- [ ] Mother with hx of type 2 diabetes
- [ ] Father with hx of high BP
- [ ] Both mother and maternal aunt with hx of gallstone disease

Social Hx

- [ ] Heavy alcohol use
- [ ] 5-6 drinks daily on weekends
- [ ] Last alcoholic beverage 5 days ago
- [ ] No recreational drugs
- [ ] Does not smoke
- [ ] Sexually active with boyfriend only
- [ ] Uses condoms
- [ ] No history of STDs

Physical Examination

- [ ] Washed hands prior to examination
- [ ] Inspected of abdomen
- [ ] Auscultated 4 quadrants + epigastric
- [ ] Percussed 4 quadrants + epigastric
- [ ] Palpated 4 quadrants
    - [ ] + voluntary guarding
    - [ ] + tenderness in RUQ, epigastrium, and LUQ
    - [ ] No rebound tenderness
- [ ] Assessed liver and spleen span
- [ ] Inspected skin for ecchymotic discoloration
- [ ] Inspected sclera
- [ ] Assessed rebound tenderness
- [ ] Tested for Murphy's sign: Murphy's sign is absent

Patient Note

History

CC: 31 yo F c/o severe abdominal pain for the past 5 hours.

HPI: Sudden onset. 10/10 severity. constant and dull. LUQ and RUQ, radiating to the back. Aspirin did not relieve symptoms. Leaning forward helps alleviate the pain and laying supine exacerbates it. She had 3 episodes of non-bloody, non-bilious emesis. No recent sick contacts.

ROS: + Persistent nausea for several hours,. Denies fever, chills, diarrhea, cough, chest pain, dyspnea, and dark stools. Pain is not related to food intake.

PMH: similar symptoms 2 yrs ago, admitted to ICU, h/o frequent UTIs, NKDA. No new medications and no herbal medications. Uses ASA regularly. No h/o DM.

FHx: mother has type 2 diabetes, gallstone disease; father has HTN, maternal aunt w/ gallstone disease

SHx: sexually active, monogamous, regular condom use, no STDs, pt drinks 5-6 drinks daily on weekends, no recreational drug use, no tobacco use.

Physical Exam

T 101.0 F; BP102/60 mm Hg; pulse 109/min; respirations 27/min

GA: alert, conscious, and coherent; anxious and uncomfortable; in moderate distress

HEENT: no scleral icterus

Abd: No scars, bruises, or distention; BS + in 4Q; tympanic in all 4 quadrants and epigastric area; diffusely tender in epigastrium, RUQ, and LUQ, voluntary guarding; no rebound tenderness; no hepatosplenomegaly, bowel sounds present. Negative Murphy

Skin: No jaundice; negative Cullen and Grey Turner sign

Data Interpretation

DIAGNOSIS 1: ACUTE PANCREATITIS

History Findings	Physical Exam Findings
Sudden onset of upper abdominal pain	Tachycardia
Constant, dull	Fever
Radiation to back, alleviated by leaning forward	Tachypnea
Family h/o gallstone disease	Voluntary guarding
Heavy alcohol use	Tenderness in RUQ, epigastrium, and LUQ
Three episodes of vomiting	
Persistent nausea for several hours	

DIAGNOSIS 2: CHOLECYSTITIS

History Findings	Physical Exam Findings
Sudden onset of upper abdominal pain	Tachycardic 109/min
Constant	Fever
Family h/o gallstone disease	RUQ and epigastric tenderness
Three episodes of vomiting	Voluntary guarding
Persistent nausea	

DIAGNOSIS 3: PEPTIC ULCER DISEASE

History Findings	Physical Exam Findings
Sudden onset of constant upper abdominal pain	Tachycardia
Heavy alcohol use	Diffusely tender in upper abdomen
NSAID use	Guarding
Nausea and vomiting	

Diagnostic Studies

Rectal exam: fecal occult blood

Serum electrolytes, CBC with diff

Amylase

Lipase

AST, ALT, glucose

Abdominal ultrasound

Esophagogastroduodenoscopy

Case Tips and Possible Alternatives

Critical Findings	Case Variations DDX	Important to Communicate
☐ 10/10 abdominal pain **radiating to the back** ☐ **Leaning forward** alleviates pain ☐ T: 101 F, BP **102/60** mmHg	☐ Large bowel obstruction (older adults, chronic constipation, living in an institutionalized setting) ☐ Cholangitis (usually age 50–60, fever with chills, RUQ pain and jaundice)	☐ Nothing by mouth (important to prep the patient about what will happen next) ☐ Alcohol consumption (binge drinking in relation to the possible diagnosis ☐ Diet (triglyceride control, etc.)
Note: For a patient in severe pain, acknowledge the urgency to find a solution and provide care without promising things you will not be able to deliver (false promises). Also, be quick but precise in your questions and physical exam.		

CASE 11: CHRONIC DIARRHEA

Doorway Information

Opening Scenario

Bernice Roth is a 30-year-old woman who presents with complaints of recurrent diarrheal episodes for the past year.

Vital Signs

T 37.9 C (100.2 F)

BP 128/82 mm Hg

Pulse 80/min

Respirations 16/min

Examinee Tasks

1. Obtain a focused history.

2. Perform a relevant physical exam. Do not perform rectal, pelvic, genitourinary, or corneal reflex exam.

3. Discuss your initial diagnostic impression and your workup plan with the patient.

4. After leaving the room, complete your Patient Note.

Communication and Interpersonal Skills Checklist

Fostering the Relationship	Gathering Information	Providing Information
☐ Knocked	☐ Elicited chief complaint	☐ Summarized significant information
☐ Introduced self	☐ Established timeline of patient's CC	☐ Provided diagnostic impression
☐ Clarified role	☐ Used open-ended question	☐ Justified diagnosis with evidence from encounter
☐ Was properly groomed	☐ Used non-leading questions	☐ Assessed patient's need for additional information
☐ Made eye contact	☐ Used closed-ended questions	☐ Encouraged and answered questions
☐ Maintained appropriate distance	☐ Asked one question at a time	☐ Assessed patient's comprehension of probable illness
☐ Displayed confident manner	☐ Did not use medical jargon	
☐ Showed care and concern	☐ Appropriately used "continuers"	
☐ Was respectful and nonjudgmental	☐ Paraphrased	
☐ Established patient's preferred title	☐ Appropriately used transitions	
☐ Used proper draping	☐ Elicited additional concerns	
☐ Focused on patient	☐ Assessed impact on patient's life	
☐ Did not interrupt patient	☐ Checked for patient understanding	
☐ Maintained appropriate and responsive body language		

Making Decisions	Supporting Emotions
☐ Clearly stated next steps in management	☐ Actively listened and validated patient's expectations
☐ **Counseled** patient	☐ Showed empathy and used appropriate reassurances
☐ Agreed to **mutual plan** of action	☐ Inquired about patient's support system
	☐ Managed the **challenge** (here, patient asked, "Can you help?")

History and Physical Examination Checklist

HPI

- ☐ Recurrent episodes of diarrhea
- ☐ Duration: 1 year
- ☐ Waxes and wanes
- ☐ 10-20 bowel movements per day when most frequent
- ☐ Fecal incontinence (finds stool in underwear)
- ☐ Blood
    - ☐ Occasionally
    - ☐ Mixed with stool
- ☐ Large amounts of mucus
- ☐ Abdominal pain
    - ☐ Lower abdomen
    - ☐ 4/10 intensity
    - ☐ Crampy
    - ☐ No radiation
- ☐ Intermittent fevers
- ☐ Unintended 20lbs. loss in the last 12 months
- ☐ Fatigue
- ☐ Intermittent joint pain
    - ☐ Knees
- ☐ No visual changes
- ☐ No red eyes
- ☐ No skin rashes or pallor
- ☐ No known sick contacts
- ☐ No post prandial bloating
- ☐ No oral ulcers
- ☐ No steatorrhea or tenesmus
- ☐ Recent travel to Israel before onset of symptoms

PMH

- ☐ Perianal fistula
    - ☐ Repaired 1.5 years ago
- ☐ Meds: no prescription meds, no OTC
- ☐ NKDA

Family Hx

- ☐ Uncle had "problem with his intestines," which required surgery and resection
- ☐ No history of colon cancer

Social Hx

- ☐ Full time rabbinical student
- ☐ Sexually active and monogamous with husband
- ☐ Has 2 healthy children
- ☐ No drugs
- ☐ No smoking
- ☐ No alcohol use

Physical Examination

- ☐ Washed hands prior to examination
- ☐ Inspected abdomen
- ☐ Auscultated abdomen in 4 quadrants
- ☐ Percussed abdomen in all 4 quadrants
- ☐ Lightly palpated abdomen in all 4 quadrants
- ☐ Deeply palpated abdomen in all 4 quadrants
    - ☐ Mildly tender to palpation in the RLQ
    - ☐ No rebound tenderness
    - ☐ No guarding
- ☐ Inspected eyes for evidence of uveitis and episcleritis
- ☐ Examined oral mucosa
- ☐ Inspected skin for lesions and pallor
- ☐ Examined joints for evidence of inflammation

Patient Note

History

CC: 30 yo F c/o recurrent diarrheal episodes for the past year.

HPI: The diarrhea occasionally contains gross blood and mucus. She can have as many as 10-20 BMs daily with some fecal incontinence, a/w crampy lower abd pain w/o radiation. Recently traveled to Israel.

ROS: Positive for occasional fever, fatigue, 20 lb. unintended weight loss in the last year, and intermittent joint pain affecting knees particularly. No pallor, rashes, visual changes, red eyes, oral ulcers, postprandial bloating, steatorrhea, tenesmus, odynophagia, or dysphagia.

PMH: h/o perianal fistula

Allergies: no known drug allergies

Medications: no Rx, OTC medications, or supplements

FH: Uncle had GI illness with "partial gut resection." No h/o colon cancer in family

SH: no EtOH/cig/drug use

Married, has 2 healthy children. Rabbinic student

Physical Examination

VS: T 100.2 F, BP 128/82 mm Hg, pulse 80/min, respirations 16/min

GA: thin and pale, NAD

Skin: No lesions or pallor noted

Abd: BS (+) × 4Q; tympanic × 4Q; no tenderness to palpation except mild tenderness in RLQ, no guarding or rebound tenderness, no palpable masses, non distended.

Ext: no effusion/inflammation in joints

Eyes: No redness or conjunctiva pallor

Oropharynx: moist mucous membranes, no oral ulcers

Data Interpretation

DIAGNOSIS 1. CROHN DISEASE

History Findings	Physical Exam Findings
Diarrhea × 1 yr; 10–20 BMs/day w/occasional gross blood and mucus	Fever
Abdominal cramping	Mild tenderness to palpation RLQ
h/o fecal incontinence	
h/o perianal fistula	
20-lb weight loss	
h/o fever and arthralgias	
Age	
FHx of GI illness: uncle w/"partial gut resection"	

DIAGNOSIS 2. ULCERATIVE COLITIS

History Findings	Physical Exam Findings
Diarrhea × 1 yr, 10–20 BMs/day w/bloody stools	Fever
h/o fecal incontinence	Mild tenderness to palpation RLQ
20-lb weight loss	
Fever	
Arthralgias	
FHx of GI illness: uncle w/"partial gut resection"	

DIAGNOSIS 3. CHRONIC INFECTIOUS DIARRHEA (AMEBIASIS, YERSINIOSIS)

History Findings	Physical Exam Findings
Diarrhea × 1 yr, 10–20 BMs/day w/ bloody stools	Fever
	Mild tenderness to palpation RLQ
h/o fecal incontinence	
h/o fever	

Diagnostic Studies

Rectal exam

– Stool culture. Stool assays: FOB, ova and parasite. Leukocytes. Stool antigen for *E. histolytica.*

– Fecal lactoferrin and calprotectin levels

– CBC w/diff., ESR, CRP, serum albumin

– ASCA, pANCA

– Electrolytes

– Endoscopy, colonoscopy

– Abd x-ray

– Endoscopy

– Abd x-ray

Case Tips and Possible Alternatives

Critical Findings	Case Variations DDX	Important to Communicate
☐ Diarrhea × 1 year ☐ Stools with mucus and occasionally blood ☐ Fecal incontinence ☐ **Weight loss** ☐ **Joint pain** ☐ Recent travel to Israel	☐ Irritable bowel syndrome (altered bowel habits: constipation and diarrhea, abdominal pain can be precipitated by meals, defecation improves pain, no weight loss) ☐ Celiac disease (oily, frothy watery stools, flatulence, weakness, fatigue, anemia)	☐ Implications of a chronic illness, new lifestyle, diet changes, support groups, etc. ☐ Next steps ☐ Expectations management ☐ How to deal with flare-ups as well as signs and symptoms that require medical attention

Note: Patients who have chronic conditions tend to develop a change in their general appearance. Noting the patient's pallor, body habitus, tone of voice, etc. during the interview can provide clues and an idea about the severity of disease.

CASE 12: ABDOMINAL PAIN AND YELLOW SKIN

Doorway Information

Opening Scenario

Jerry Matthews is a 55-year-old man who presents because of worsening abdominal pain and yellow skin for the past 2 weeks.

Vital Signs

T 37.1 C (98.8 F)

BP 118/72 mm Hg

Pulse 95/min

Respirations 14/min

Examinee Tasks

1. Obtain a focused history.

2. Perform a relevant physical exam. Do not perform rectal, pelvic, genitourinary, or corneal reflex exam.

3. Discuss your initial diagnostic impression and your workup plan with the patient.

4. After leaving the room, complete your Patient Note on the given form.

Communication and Interpersonal Skills Checklist

Fostering the Relationship	Gathering Information	Providing Information
☐ Knocked	☐ Elicited chief complaint	☐ Summarized significant information
☐ Introduced self	☐ Established timeline of patient's CC	☐ Provided diagnostic impression
☐ Clarified role	☐ Used open-ended question	☐ Justified diagnosis with evidence from encounter
☐ Was properly groomed	☐ Used non-leading questions	☐ Assessed patient's need for additional information
☐ Made eye contact	☐ Used closed-ended questions	☐ Encouraged and answered questions
☐ Maintained appropriate distance	☐ Asked one question at a time	☐ Assessed patient's comprehension of probable illness
☐ Displayed confident manner	☐ Did not use medical jargon	
☐ Showed care and concern	☐ Appropriately used "continuers"	
☐ Was respectful and nonjudgmental	☐ Paraphrased	
☐ Established patient's preferred title	☐ Appropriately used transitions	
☐ Used proper draping	☐ Elicited additional concerns	
☐ Focused on patient	☐ Assessed impact on patient's life	
☐ Did not interrupt patient	☐ Checked for patient understanding	
☐ Maintained appropriate and responsive body language		

Making Decisions	Supporting Emotions
☐ Clearly stated next steps in management	☐ Actively listened and validated patient's expectations
☐ **Counseled** patient	☐ Showed empathy and used appropriate reassurances
☐ Agreed to **mutual plan** of action	☐ Inquired about patient's support system
	☐ Managed the **challenge** (here; patient asked, "This is because of my drinking, isn't it?")

History and Physical Examination Checklist

HPI

- ☐ Abdominal pain
  - ☐ Duration: 2 weeks
  - ☐ Progressively worsening
  - ☐ RUQ
  - ☐ Dull
  - ☐ 5/10 intensity
  - ☐ Constant
  - ☐ No radiation
- ☐ Jaundice
- ☐ Dark urine
- ☐ Light colored stools
- ☐ Fatigue
- ☐ No nausea
- ☐ No vomiting or diarrhea
- ☐ No diaphoresis or malaise
- ☐ No fever
- ☐ No bruising
- ☐ No rectal bleeding or hematemesis
- ☐ No history of confusion
- ☐ No history of distended abdomen
- ☐ No muscle weakness
- ☐ 20 lb weight loss
  - ☐ Over the last 2 mos
  - ☐ Doesn't feel hungry
  - ☐ Drinks instead

PMH

- ☐ History of degenerative joint disease
  - ☐ Knees
  - ☐ Takes large amounts of acetaminophen for the pain
- ☐ Meds: no prescription meds, OTC acetaminophen
- ☐ NKDA

Family Hx

- ☐ No significant family history
- ☐ Except an uncle who died of liver problems
- ☐ Not been around anyone sick recently

Social Hx

- ☐ Currently unemployed
- ☐ Lives in homeless shelter
- ☐ Denies smoking
- ☐ Alcohol use
  - ☐ Heavy drinker
  - ☐ Past 5-10 years
  - ☐ Just finished a week-long binge
- ☐ Denies current drug use
  - ☐ Used to inject heroin
- ☐ Not current sexually active
  - ☐ Numerous past sexual partners
  - ☐ Does not use condoms regularly
  - ☐ Unsure of HIV status
- ☐ No recent travel

Physical Examination

- ☐ Washed hands prior to examination
- ☐ Checked for scleral icterus (+)
- ☐ Checked for jaundice (+)
- ☐ Inspected mucous membranes (dry)
- ☐ Performed MMSE
- ☐ Inspected abdomen
  - ☐ Non-distended
- ☐ Auscultated abdomen in all 4 quadrants
- ☐ Percussed abdomen in all 4 quadrants
  - ☐ Measured liver span
    - ☐ Liver edge is palpable 6-7 cm below costal margin
- ☐ Lightly palpated abdomen in all 4 quadrants

- ☐ Deeply palpated abdomen in all non-tender quadrants
  - ☐ Tenderness in RUQ
- ☐ Checked for splenomegaly
  - ☐ Spleen is not palpable
- ☐ Checked for presence of Murphy sign (−)
- ☐ Checked for rebound tenderness
- ☐ Examined for ascites
  - ☐ No shifting dullness or fluid wave
- ☐ Checked extremities for edema
- ☐ Checked palms for erythema
- ☐ Checked skin for spider angiomata

Patient Note

History

CC: 55 yo M c/o worsening abdominal pain and yellow skin for the past 2 weeks.

HPI: The pain is located in the RUQ, is 5/10, dull, constant, and non-radiating. He also notes a 2 month history of 20 lb weight loss. He also reports a history of degenerative joint disease of the knees and has been taking acetaminophen on a daily basis.

ROS: Positive for anorexia, fatigue, choluria, and acholic stools. Denies confusion, vomiting, diarrhea, abd. distention, diaphoresis, malaise, muscle weakness or fever.

PMH: no prior occurrences of similar event, knee osteoarthritis, h/o alcoholism × 5–10 yrs

Allergies: NKDA

Medications: No Rx, OTC acetaminophen

FH: Uncle: liver failure

SH: Homeless, lives in shelter, unemployed. Non-smoker. Heavy alcohol use, last drink today after week long binge. Past h/o IVDU (heroin). Not currently sexually active. Unsure of HIV status, multiple sexual partners without condoms

Physical Examination

VS: T 37.1 C (98.8 F), BP 118/72 mm Hg, pulse 95/min, respirations 14/min

Gen: malnourished, jaundiced, appears older than stated age, NAD

HEENT: scleral icterus, dry mucous membranes

Abd: BS (+) × 4Q; tympanic to percussion × 4Q, marked hepatomegaly. No splenomegaly. No distention. No tenderness except on RUQ. No guarding, rebound, or Murphy's sign. No shifting dullness or fluid wave

Skin: no lesions or spider angiomata

Ext: no palmar erythema, no edema

Data Interpretation

DIAGNOSIS 1. ALCOHOLIC HEPATITIS

History Findings	Physical Exam Findings
Jaundice	Malnourished, NAD
RUQ pain	Jaundice, scleral icterus
Choluria, acholic stools	RUQ tenderness
h/o alcoholism	No Murphy's sign
Homeless, lives in shelter, unemployed	Tender hepatomegaly
Fatigue	

Diagnosis 2. Viral Hepatitis (B or C)

History Findings	Physical Exam Findings
Jaundice	Malnourished, NAD
Weight loss, malaise, anorexia	Jaundice, scleral icterus
Choluria, acholic stools	No Murphy's sign
Homeless, lives in shelter	RUQ tenderness
Past h/o IVDU (heroin)	Hepatomegaly
Multiple sexual partners without condoms	

Diagnosis 3. Acetaminophen Toxicity

History Findings	Physical Exam Findings
Jaundice	NAD
Choluria, acholic stools	Jaundice, scleral icterus
RUQ pain	RUQ tenderness
Medications: acetaminophen	No Murphy's sign
Anorexia	Hepatomegaly

Diagnostic Studies

CBC w/ differential

AST, ALT, alkaline phosphatase, total bilirubin, direct bilirubin, indirect bilirubin, albumin, total protein

PT/INR, PTT

HCV antibody, HCV PCR, HBsAg, HBsAb, HBV core Ab IgM

Acetaminophen level

RUQ U/S

Case Tips and Possible Alternatives

Critical Findings	Case Variations DDX	Important to Communicate
☐ Progressively worsening RUQ pain of 2 weeks duration ☐ Jaundice ☐ Weight loss ☐ Homeless ☐ Alcoholism ☐ Heavy use of acetaminophen	☐ Acalculous cholecystitis (HIV, prolonged fasting, abdominal pain in RUQ that might radiate to right shoulder) ☐ Cholelithiasis (female, reproductive age, European descent, asymptomatic or biliary colic)	☐ Addressing current problem: alcohol intake/cessation, diet, continuing medical treatment ☐ Addressing chronic problems: homelessness, alcoholism. ☐ Addressing acetaminophen use
Note: Patients experiencing homelessness have a myriad of health issues that usually become secondary to daily struggles of finding, food, shelter and clothing. They have an unusual health burden that is related to physical issues, mental health challenges, and substance abuse.		

CASE 13: COUGH

Doorway Information

Opening Scenario

Paul Lambert is a 66-year-old man who presents to the ER complaining of worsening cough.

Vital Signs

T 38.3 C (101.0 F)

BP 146/90 mm Hg

Pulse 107/min

Respirations 28/min

SpO2 90% on room air

Examinee Tasks

1. Obtain a focused history.

2. Perform a relevant physical exam. Do not perform rectal, pelvic, genitourinary, or corneal reflex exam.

3. Discuss your initial diagnostic impression and your workup plan with the patient.

4. After leaving the room, complete your Patient Note on the given form.

Communication and Interpersonal Skills Checklist

Fostering the Relationship	Gathering Information	Providing Information
☐ Knocked	☐ Elicited chief complaint	☐ Summarized significant information
☐ Introduced self	☐ Established timeline of patient's CC	☐ Provided diagnostic impression
☐ Clarified role	☐ Used open-ended question	☐ Justified diagnosis with evidence from encounter
☐ Was properly groomed	☐ Used non-leading questions	☐ Assessed patient's need for additional information
☐ Made eye contact	☐ Used closed-ended questions	☐ Encouraged and answered questions
☐ Maintained appropriate distance	☐ Asked one question at a time	☐ Assessed patient's comprehension of probable illness
☐ Displayed confident manner	☐ Did not use medical jargon	
☐ Showed care and concern	☐ Appropriately used "continuers"	
☐ Was respectful and nonjudgmental	☐ Paraphrased	
☐ Established patient's preferred title	☐ Appropriately used transitions	
☐ Used proper draping	☐ Elicited additional concerns	
☐ Focused on patient	☐ Assessed impact on patient's life	
☐ Did not interrupt patient	☐ Checked for patient understanding	
☐ Maintained appropriate and responsive body language		

Making Decisions	Supporting Emotions
☐ Clearly stated next steps in management	☐ Actively listened and validated patient's expectations
☐ **Counseled** patient	☐ Showed empathy and used appropriate reassurances
☐ Agreed to **mutual plan** of action	☐ Inquired about patient's support system
	☐ Managed the **challenge** (here; patient asked, "Is it serious?")

History and Physical Examination Checklist

HPI

- ☐ Chronic cough
  - ☐ Duration: 6 mos
  - ☐ Productive
    - ☐ 1 teaspoonful
- ☐ Cough worse over past 3 days
  - ☐ Currently a greenish-yellow sputum
  - ☐ Blood streaks on sputum
- ☐ Shortness of breath
  - ☐ When climbing up stairs
- ☐ Fever
  - ☐ Low grade
- ☐ No chills
- ☐ No night sweats
- ☐ Wheezing
  - ☐ Intermittent
  - ☐ Requires albuterol inhaler
- ☐ No chest pain
- ☐ No sick contacts
- ☐ No travel
- ☐ No dysphonia
- ☐ No halitosis
- ☐ Fatigue
- ☐ No bone pain
- ☐ Usual exercise tolerance lower
- ☐ Weight loss
  - ☐ 20 lbs
  - ☐ Over 3 mos

PMH

- ☐ COPD
- ☐ 2 previous episodes of pneumonia
  - ☐ Treated
  - ☐ 1 required hospitalization
- ☐ Hypertension
- ☐ No surgery
- ☐ Meds
  - ☐ Atenolol
  - ☐ Ipratropium inhaler daily
  - ☐ Albuterol (as needed)
- ☐ NKDA

Family Hx

- ☐ No significant family history
- ☐ Not been around anyone sick recently

Social Hx

- ☐ 40-pack-year hx of smoking tobacco
  - ☐ Stopped smoking 3 days ago (due to illness)
- ☐ No alcohol use
- ☐ No drug use
- ☐ Retired postal worker

Physical Examination

- ☐ Washed hands prior to examination
- ☐ Assessed the patient for respiratory distress
- ☐ Performed a lymph node exam of the neck
- ☐ Assessed neck for JVD
- ☐ Performed inspection of chest
  - ☐ Chest wall appears symmetrical
- ☐ Performed percussion of lungs
- ☐ Assessed for tactile fremitus
  - ☐ Decreased tactile fremitus
- ☐ Auscultated lungs
  - ☐ Coughs when asked to breathe deeply
  - ☐ Scattered expiratory wheezes bilaterally, but no crackles or rales
- ☐ Examined extremities for cyanosis/clubbing/edema
- ☐ Examined oropharynx
- ☐ Performed cardiac auscultation
- ☐ Assessed PMI

Patient Note

History

CC: 66 yo M c/o worsening cough.

HPI: Past medical history notable for COPD with chronic bronchitis characterized by productive cough, presents to the ED with a worsening cough × 3 days. The cough is now productive of increasing amounts of greenish-yellow sputum, sometimes blood-tinged, and is aggravated by deep breathing, associated intermittent chest tightness and wheezing with increased use of his albuterol inhaler and increased DOE. He denies sick contacts, recent travel, or chest pain.

ROS: + Chronic fatigue, + low grade fevers, + 20lb. unintended weight loss/3 mos, denies chest pain, shaking chills, night sweats, swelling of LE, bone pain, dystonia, and dysphagia.

PMH: h/o pneumonia × 2, COPD, HTN, no surgeries

Allergies: NKDA

Meds: atenolol, ipratropium, albuterol prn

FHx: no major illness

S Hx: 40 pack/year; no h/o EtOH or rec drugs

Physical Exam

BP 146/90 mm Hg, pulse 107/min, T 38.3 C (101.0 F) respirations 28/min, SpO2: 90% on RA

Gen: appears anxious, uncomfortable, and in mild respiratory distress

Oropharynx: no lesions or blood present

Neck: no lymphadenopathy or JVD

Chest: symmetric, no dullness to percussion; scattered expiratory wheezes bilaterally, no rales or rhonchi, decreased fremitus throughout.

CV: normal S1, S2, no m/r/g, non-displaced PMI

Ext: no clubbing, cyanosis, or edema

Data Interpretation

Diagnosis 1. Lung Cancer

History Findings	Physical Exam Findings
Worsening cough	Pulse 107/min, respirations 28/min, T: 38.3 C (101.0 F), SpO2: 90% RA
DOE	Evidence of respiratory distress
Hemoptysis	Scattered expiratory wheezes
20 lb weight loss	Decreased fremitus
Chronic fatigue	
40 pack/year smoking history	

DIAGNOSIS 2. PNEUMONIA

History Findings	Physical Exam Findings
Worsening cough with increased sputum production	Pulse 107/min, respirations 28/min, T: 38.3 C (101.0 F), SpO2: 90% RA
Low grade fever	Evidence of respiratory distress
DOE	Expiratory wheezes on chest exam
Intermittent chest tightness	
40-pack-year smoking history	
Wheezing	
h/o COPD	
h/o pneumonia × 2	

DIAGNOSIS 3. COPD EXACERBATION

History Findings	Physical Exam Findings
Worsening cough w/increased sputum production	pulse 107/min, respirations 28/min, T: 38.3 C (101.0 F), SpO2: 90% RA
Increased DOE	Evidence of respiratory distress
Fever	Expiratory wheezes on chest exam
h/o COPD with increased rescue inhaler use	Overall decreased tactile fremitus
Intermittent chest tightness	Lack of dullness to percussion
Wheezing	
Fatigue	
40-pack-year smoking history	

Diagnostic Studies

CXR

Sputum Gram stain & culture

CBC w/ diff

Arterial blood gas

Blood cultures

EKG

Echo

Chest CT

Case Tips and Possible Alternatives

Critical Findings	Case Variations DDX	Important to Communicate
☐ Productive cough >6 months ☐ Hemoptysis ☐ Weight loss ☐ Short of breath going up stairs ☐ 40-pack-year smoking	☐ Congestive heart failure (exertional dyspnea, orthopnea, cyanosis, pallor, edema) ☐ Pulmonary embolism (short of breath, pleuritic pain, productive cough, hemoptysis)	☐ Maintaining tobacco cessation ☐ Preparing the patient for the possibility of bad news (cancer diagnosis)
Note: It is very hard to quitting smoking, so physicians must be understanding. Don't impose judgment, and don't shame the patient into changing behavior.		

CASE 14: BLOOD IN URINE

Doorway Information

Opening Scenario

Matthew Howe is a 60 year-old man who comes to your office because of intermittent blood in his urine over the past 1 month.

Vital Signs

T 37 C (98.6 F)

BP 150/95 mm Hg

Pulse 62/min

Respirations 14/min

Examinee Tasks

1. Obtain a pertinent history.

2. Perform a relevant physical examination. Do not perform a pelvic/genital, corneal reflex, or rectal examination.

3. Discuss your impressions and any initial plans with the patient.

4. After leaving the room, complete your Patient Note.

Communication and Interpersonal Skills Checklist

Fostering the Relationship	Gathering Information	Providing Information
☐ Knocked	☐ Elicited chief complaint	☐ Summarized significant information
☐ Introduced self	☐ Established timeline of patient's CC	☐ Provided diagnostic impression
☐ Clarified role	☐ Used open-ended question	☐ Justified diagnosis with evidence from encounter
☐ Was properly groomed	☐ Used non-leading questions	☐ Assessed patient's need for additional information
☐ Made eye contact	☐ Used closed-ended questions	☐ Encouraged and answered questions
☐ Maintained appropriate distance	☐ Asked one question at a time	☐ Assessed patient's comprehension of probable illness
☐ Displayed confident manner	☐ Did not use medical jargon	
☐ Showed care and concern	☐ Appropriately used "continuers"	
☐ Was respectful and nonjudgmental	☐ Paraphrased	
☐ Established patient's preferred title	☐ Appropriately used transitions	
☐ Used proper draping	☐ Elicited additional concerns	
☐ Focused on patient	☐ Assessed impact on patient's life	
☐ Did not interrupt patient	☐ Checked for patient understanding	
☐ Maintained appropriate and responsive body language		

Making Decisions	Supporting Emotions
☐ Clearly stated next steps in management	☐ Actively listened and validated patient's expectations
☐ **Counseled** patient	☐ Showed empathy and used appropriate reassurances
☐ Agreed to **mutual plan** of action	☐ Inquired about patient's support system
	☐ Managed the **challenge** (here; patient asked, "is it cancer?")

History and Physical Examination Checklist

HPI

- ☐ Hematuria
- ☐ Duration: 1 month
- ☐ 3 episodes
- ☐ Blood present throughout micturition
- ☐ No pain
- ☐ Increased urinary frequency
- ☐ Nocturia 3-4 times per night
- ☐ Weak stream
- ☐ Incomplete voiding
- ☐ Weight loss
- ☐ No fever or chills
- ☐ No fatigue
- ☐ No Hx of peripheral or periorbital edema
- ☐ No dysuria
- ☐ No oliguria
- ☐ No recent trauma
- ☐ Sore throat 6 wks ago
- ☐ No recent travel

PMH

- ☐ HTN (controlled)
- ☐ Nephrolithiasis (5 years ago) treated with lithotripsy
- ☐ No joint pain
- ☐ No skin rashes
- ☐ Meds: aspirin and amlodipine
- ☐ NKDA

Family Hx

- ☐ Father had prostate cancer

Social Hx

- ☐ No alcohol, no drugs
- ☐ Quit smoking
- ☐ Previous 2 years × 30 pack/yr hx of tobacco
- ☐ Married, monogamous, no hx of STDs
- ☐ Profession is law, no factory work
- ☐ No exposure to toxins

Physical Examination

- ☐ Washed hands prior to examination
- ☐ Inspected skin
- ☐ Inspected abdomen
- ☐ Auscultated abdomen in 4 quadrants
- ☐ Percussed abdomen in 4 quadrants
- ☐ Palpated abdomen in 4 quadrants
- ☐ Examined for costovertebral angle tenderness
- ☐ Auscultated lungs
- ☐ Checked for peripheral edema
- ☐ Checked for peri-orbital edema
- ☐ Inspected oropharynx
- ☐ Palpated lymph nodes

Patient Note

History

CC: 60 yo M c/o intermittent blood in his urine over the past 1 month.

HPI: 3 episodes in last month. The episodes are painless. The blood is seen in the urine throughout the episodes of micturition. He also had a sore throat 6 weeks ago and lost some weight. He has a h/o well-controlled HTN. He has no known toxic exposures.

ROS: Positive for urinary frequency, nocturia, weak stream, and feeling of incomplete voiding for the past 3-4 mos. Denies fever, chills, dysuria, oliguria, edema, fatigue, joint pain nor pain anywhere else in his body, skin rashes.

PMH: HTN, 1 episode of nephrolithiasis 5 years ago treated with lithotripsy; no recent trauma

Medications: amlodipine, aspirin

Allergies: NKDA

Family Hx: father had prostate cancer

Social Hx: 60-pack-year smoking history (quit 10 years ago), no EtOH, married, monogamous, works as a lawyer, no recent travel

---

Physical Exam

Vitals: T 98.6 F, BP 150/95 mm Hg, pulse 62/min, R 14/min

General: comfortable, no acute distress

Skin: no rashes

HEENT: oropharynx without lesions or tonsillar exudates; no peri-orbital edema

Chest: clear to auscultation, no wheezes, rales, or rhonchi b/l

Abd: +BS x4 quadrants, tympanic to percussion x4 quadrants, non-tender, non-distended, no masses palpated, no organomegaly

Back: no costovertebral angle tenderness

Extremities no peripheral edema

Lymph nodes: no palpable nodes in neck, axilla, or groin

Data Interpretation

DIAGNOSIS 1. BLADDER CANCER

History Findings	Physical Exam Findings
Painless hematuria	No fever
Blood present throughout micturition	No tenderness on palpation or abdominal masses
Polyuria and increased urgency	
60 pack year smoking history	
Weight loss	

DIAGNOSIS 2. POST-STREPTOCOCCAL GLOMERULONEPHRITIS (GN)

History Findings	Physical Exam Findings
Gross hematuria	Elevated BP
Hypertension	
Recent pharyngitis	

DIAGNOSIS 3. PROSTATE CANCER

History Findings	Physical Exam Findings
Gross hematuria	No fever
Nocturia	No tenderness on palpation or abdominal masses
Polyuria and increased urgency	
Family history of prostate cancer	
Weight loss	

Diagnostic Studies

Prostate exam

Antistreptolysin O titer; complement levels

Urinalysis/urine culture

PSA

BUN, creatinine

Urine cytology

Cystoscopy

Trans-rectal ultrasound

Case Tips and Possible Alternatives

Critical Findings	Case Variations DDX	Important to Communicate
☐ **Painless, episodic, gross** hematuria of 1 month duration ☐ 60-pack-year **smoking** Hx. ☐ Weight loss	☐ UTI in males (dysuria, nocturia, hematuria, comorbid conditions like diabetes, prostatitis, epididymitis, etc.)	☐ Preparing the patient for the possibility of bad news (cancer Dx.) ☐ Continuing smoking cessation ☐ Next steps and expectations
Note: Weight loss, fatigue, fever are nonspecific signs. Since symptoms can be important predictors for more severe disease, ask the patient to be specific: clarify when symptoms first started, clarify what "fatigue" means, and explain the weight loss in more detail.		

CASE 15: PEDIATRIC DIARRHEA

Doorway Information

Opening Scenario

Margaret Swanson is the mother of a 1-year-old son calling your office because he has diarrhea.

Vital Signs

Child is not available for physical exam

Examinee Tasks

1. Obtain a focused history.

2. There is no physical exam in this case.

3. Discuss your initial diagnostic impression and your workup plan with the mother.

4. After leaving the room, complete your Patient Note on the given form.

Communication and Interpersonal Skills Checklist

Fostering the Relationship	Gathering Information	Providing Information
☐ Introduced self ☐ Clarified role ☐ Displayed confident manner ☐ Showed care and concern ☐ Was respectful and nonjudgmental ☐ Established preferred title ☐ Did not interrupt	☐ Elicited chief complaint ☐ Established timeline of patient's CC ☐ Used open-ended question ☐ Used non-leading questions ☐ Used closed-ended questions ☐ Asked one question at a time ☐ Did not use medical jargon ☐ Appropriately used "continuers" ☐ Paraphrased ☐ Appropriately used transitions ☐ Elicited additional concerns ☐ Assessed impact on patient's life ☐ Checked for understanding	☐ Summarized significant information ☐ Provided diagnostic impression ☐ Justified diagnosis with evidence from encounter ☐ Assessed need for additional information ☐ Encouraged and answered questions ☐ Assessed comprehension of probable illness

Making Decisions	Supporting Emotions
☐ Clearly stated next steps in management ☐ **Counseled** relative ☐ Agreed to **mutual plan** of action	☐ Actively listened and validated expectations ☐ Showed empathy and used appropriate reassurances ☐ Inquired about patient's support system ☐ Managed the **challenge** (here; mother asked, "will he require IV fluids?")

History and Physical Examination Checklist

HPI

- ☐ Diarrhea
  - ☐ Watery
  - ☐ Duration: 3 days
  - ☐ Loose stools
  - ☐ Foul smelling
  - ☐ Some blood and mucus
  - ☐ More diaper changes per day than usual
- ☐ Vomiting
  - ☐ 2 episodes
  - ☐ Non-bloody
  - ☐ Greenish
- ☐ Tried oral rehydration therapy
  - ☐ Worried child needs IV fluids
- ☐ Low grade fever
- ☐ Irritable
- ☐ No rash
- ☐ No recent dietary changes
- ☐ No tenesmus
- ☐ No appetite
- ☐ No seizures
- ☐ Difficulty feeding

PMH

- ☐ No recent illness
- ☐ Birth history is unremarkable
- ☐ Vaginal delivery at 39 weeks
- ☐ Prenatal screenings normal
- ☐ No complications in neonatal period
- ☐ No food allergies
- ☐ Appropriate growth curve
- ☐ Age appropriate vaccinations completed
- ☐ Recently began to walk and speak a few words
- ☐ No hospitalizations or surgery
- ☐ Meds: acetaminophen; no prescription meds
- ☐ NKDA

Family Hx

- ☐ No similar symptoms with family members
- ☐ No siblings
- ☐ No significant family history

Social Hx

- ☐ Recent travel to India
- ☐ Sick contacts at day care
- ☐ Unsure of HIV status

Physical Examination

No physical exam

Patient Note

History

CC: 1 yo M with diarrhea.

HPI: 3-day h/o diarrhea and episodes of non-bloody, greenish vomitus, stools are watery, loose, and foul-smelling, on oral rehydration solution, + low-grade fever, extremely irritable, + anorexia, child's playmates at the day care have also become ill, though no one in the family is affected. Recent travel to India to visit relatives. Child was healthy and active prior to onset of symptoms.

ROS: + blood and mucus on stools once or twice,. Denies rash, high fever, tenesmus, and seizures.

PMH: none

Birth Hx: unremarkable; mother had NSVD at 39 wks. and an unremarkable pre-natal course. All prenatal evaluations were reportedly normal; no complication in neonatal period.

Allergies: NKDA

Medications: pediatric acetaminophen as needed, no Rx meds

Social Hx: lives at home with his parents, no siblings

Family Hx: unremarkable

Immunization hx: up-to-date according to age

_____

Physical Exam

N/A

_____

Data Interpretation

DIAGNOSIS 1. ACUTE BACTERIAL GASTROENTERITIS

History Findings	Physical Exam Findings
Irritability	
Bloody diarrhea	
Recent travel history	
Anorexia	
Vomiting	
Fever	
Sick contacts at daycare	

DIAGNOSIS 2. ACUTE VIRAL GASTROENTERITIS

History Findings	Physical Exam Findings
Irritability	
Watery diarrhea	
Low-grade fever	
Anorexia	
Vomiting	
Daycare exposure	

DIAGNOSIS 3. GIARDIASIS

History Findings	Physical Exam Findings
Irritability	
Watery diarrhea	
Foul-smelling diarrhea	
Recent travel history	
Vomiting	

Diagnostic Studies

Physical exam of patient

CBC with differential

Serum electrolytes

Stool culture, fecal leukocytes, ova and parasites

Blood cultures

Rotavirus enzyme immunoassay

Fecal lactoferrin

Case Tips and Possible Alternatives

Critical Findings	Case Variations DDX	Important to Communicate
☐ Irritability ☐ Bloody diarrhea ☐ Travel hx ☐ Vomiting ☐ Fever ☐ **Age**	☐ Intussusception (age 6–12 months, crampy, intermittent but toxic-appearing with possible bloody diarrhea) ☐ Hemolytic uremic syndrome (prodromal illness w/ abdominal pain and diarrhea followed by hemolytic anemia, acute kidney injury and thrombocytopenia)	☐ Rehydration ☐ Warning signs for dehydration ☐ Fever management and warning signs that merit immediate medical attention
Note: Pediatric patients and older patients can dehydrate quickly. As you recommend next management steps to parents and care providers, provide clear instructions about how to keep the patient hydrated and how to watch for alarm signs/symptoms.		

CASE 16: DIZZINESS

Doorway Information

Opening Scenario

Connie Thomas is a 43-year-old woman who comes to your office complaining of dizziness.

Vital Signs

T 37.0 C (98.6 F)

BP 128/84 mm Hg

Pulse 66/min

Respirations 14/min

Examinee Tasks

1. Obtain a focused history.

2. Perform a relevant physical exam. Do not perform rectal, pelvic, genitourinary, female breast, or corneal reflex exam.

3. Discuss your initial diagnostic impression and your workup plan with the patient.

4. After leaving the room, complete your Patient Note on the given form.

Communication and Interpersonal Skills Checklist

Fostering the Relationship	Gathering Information	Providing Information
☐ Knocked	☐ Elicited chief complaint	☐ Summarized significant information
☐ Introduced self	☐ Established timeline of patient's CC	☐ Provided diagnostic impression
☐ Clarified role	☐ Used open-ended question	☐ Justified diagnosis with evidence from encounter
☐ Was properly groomed	☐ Used non-leading questions	
☐ Made eye contact	☐ Used closed-ended questions	☐ Assessed patient's need for additional information
☐ Maintained appropriate distance	☐ Asked one question at a time	☐ Encouraged and answered questions
☐ Displayed confident manner	☐ Did not use medical jargon	☐ Assessed patient's comprehension of probable illness
☐ Showed care and concern	☐ Appropriately used "continuers"	
☐ Was respectful and nonjudgmental	☐ Paraphrased	
☐ Established patient's preferred title	☐ Appropriately used transitions	
☐ Used proper draping	☐ Elicited additional concerns	
☐ Focused on patient	☐ Assessed impact on patient's life	
☐ Did not interrupt patient	☐ Checked for patient understanding	
☐ Maintained appropriate and responsive body language		

Making Decisions	Supporting Emotions
☐ Clearly stated next steps in management	☐ Actively listened and validated patient's expectations
☐ **Counseled** patient	☐ Showed empathy and used appropriate reassurances
☐ Agreed to **mutual plan** of action	☐ Inquired about patient's support system
	☐ Managed the **challenge** (here; patient has difficulty understanding you)

History and Physical Examination Checklist

HPI

- ☐ Episodic dizziness
- ☐ Duration: 6 mos
- ☐ Last episode 1 week ago
- ☐ Unsteady on feet
- ☐ Room spinning
- ☐ Spell duration: 20 minutes to a few hours
- ☐ No precipitating factor
- ☐ Relieved by lying still
- ☐ Aggravated by positional changes
- ☐ + nausea
- ☐ + vomiting
- ☐ Fluctuating hearing loss
  - ☐ Difficulty understanding speech
  - ☐ Left ear > right
  - ☐ Sensation of fullness in the ear
  - ☐ Low pitched buzz heard predominately in left ear
- ☐ No fever
- ☐ No chills
- ☐ No weakness or facial paralysis
- ☐ No sensory changes
- ☐ No paresthesias, hyperesthesia or pain
- ☐ No visual changes
- ☐ No headache
- ☐ No syncope

PMH

- ☐ No similar illness
- ☐ No history of head trauma
- ☐ History of HTN
- ☐ No hospitalizations or surgery
- ☐ Meds: atenolol and aspirin
- ☐ NKDA

Family Hx

- ☐ Father hx of stroke
- ☐ Mother hx of high cholesterol and HTN

Social Hx

- ☐ No tobacco use
- ☐ No alcohol use
- ☐ No recreational drug use
- ☐ Regular exercise
- ☐ On a healthy diet
- ☐ Single, lives alone
- ☐ Works as a web designer

Physical Examination

- ☐ Washed hands prior to examination
- ☐ Performed inspection of head
- ☐ Performed fundoscopic exam
- ☐ Performed pupillary reflex
- ☐ Assessed EOM
- ☐ Performed external ear and otoscopic exams
- ☐ Performed Weber's test
  - ☐ Sounds lateralized to the right
- ☐ Performed Rinne's test
  - ☐ Air conduction > bone conduction bilaterally
- ☐ Examined CN II–XII
- ☐ Assessed motor strength bilaterally
- ☐ Examined DTRs
- ☐ Assessed 2 modalities of sensation (light, sharp/dull)
- ☐ Assessed cerebellar function with finger-to-nose or rapid alternating movements
- ☐ Performed Romberg test
  - ☐ Negative
- ☐ Assessed gait

Patient Note

History

CC: 43 yo F c/o dizziness.

HPI: Onset 6 months ago with most recent episode occurring 1 week ago. There is no clear precipitant. The dizziness is described as the room spinning and gait unsteadiness. Episodes last from 20 minutes to a few hours and are associated with fluctuating loss of hearing, fullness and a buzzing sound all in the left ear, and sometimes nausea and vomiting. Dizziness is relieved by lying still; positional changes seem to make it worse.

ROS: positive for nausea and vomiting; negative for fever, chills, weakness or facial paralysis, sensory changes, visual changes, facial paresthesia, hyperesthesia or pain, headache, syncope

PMH: HTN, no history of head trauma

Allergies: denies

Meds: aspirin, atenolol

FH: father had a stroke, mother has HTN, HLD

SH: denies smoking, illicit drug use, and EtOH use. Single, lives alone, and works as web designer

Physical Examination

BP 128/84 mm Hg, pulse 66/min, T 37.0 C (98.6 F), Respirations 14/min

Gen: appears comfortable and NAD, speech is normal

HEENT: Normocephalic, atraumatic, no papilledema or optic disc blurring on fundoscopy, PEERLA, EOMI, TM seen; no erythema, polyps or exudates; Weber test: lateralizes to R side; Rinne test: AC > BC bilaterally

Neuro: CN II–XII intact, motor: 5/5 b/l, DTR: 2+ bilaterally: sensory system grossly intact, negative Romberg test, no intention tremor/dysmetria/gait abnormalities

Data Interpretation

DIAGNOSIS 1. MENIERE DISEASE

History Findings	Physical Exam Findings
Episodic vertigo	Weber and Rinne tests suggest sensorineural hearing loss
Lasts from 20 min to few hrs	Normal speech pattern
Tinnitus	CN II–XII intact
Fluctuating hypoacusia	Motor: 5/5 bilaterally
Ataxia during episodes	Sensory intact
Nausea and vomiting	
Aural fullness	

DIAGNOSIS 2. BENIGN PAROXYSMAL POSITIONAL VERTIGO

History Findings	Physical Exam Findings
Episodic vertigo worse with positional changes	CN II–XII intact
Ataxia during episodes	Motor: 5/5 bilaterally
Nausea, vomiting	Sensory intact

DIAGNOSIS 3. VESTIBULAR SCHWANNOMA (ACOUSTIC NEUROMA)

History Findings	Physical Exam Findings
Vertigo was gradual in onset 6 mos ago	Weber and Rinne tests suggest sensorineural hearing loss
Tinnitus and hearing loss	
Hypoacusia	
Ataxia during episodes	
Aural fullness	

Diagnostic Studies

Head MRI and CT

Dix-Hallpike test

Audiogram

RPR

Case Tips and Possible Alternatives

Critical Findings	Case Variations DDX	Important to Communicate
☐ Episodic dizziness ☐ Tinnitus ☐ **Fluctuating hypoacusia**	☐ Otosclerosis (slow, progressive, bilateral hearing loss, decade 3 of life, F > M) ☐ Presbycusis (bilateral high-frequency hearing loss, age >65)	☐ Managing tinnitus (sound therapy, relaxation techniques) ☐ Protecting hearing (avoiding loud noises, etc) ☐ Fall prevention (dizziness)
Note: Hearing loss is becoming more common, with noise exposure one of the biggest causes. Familiarize yourself with simple steps to protect hearing—especially for children and those who work in loud environments.		

CASE 17: DIFFICULTY SWALLOWING

Doorway Information

Opening Scenario

Gary Schwartz is a 52-year-old man who presents to your office complaining of difficulty swallowing.

Vital Signs

T 37.3 C (99.1 F)

BP 148/78 mm Hg

Pulse 74/min

Respirations 16/min

Examinee Tasks

1. Obtain a focused history.

2. Perform a relevant physical exam. Do not perform rectal, pelvic, genitourinary, or corneal reflex exam.

3. Discuss your initial diagnostic impression and your workup plan with the patient.

4. After leaving the room, complete your Patient Note on the given form.

Communication and Interpersonal Skills Checklist

Fostering the Relationship	Gathering Information	Providing Information
☐ Knocked	☐ Elicited chief complaint	☐ Summarized significant information
☐ Introduced self	☐ Established timeline of patient's CC	☐ Provided diagnostic impression
☐ Clarified role	☐ Used open-ended question	☐ Justified diagnosis with evidence from encounter
☐ Was properly groomed	☐ Used non-leading questions	☐ Assessed patient's need for additional information
☐ Made eye contact	☐ Used closed-ended questions	☐ Encouraged and answered questions
☐ Maintained appropriate distance	☐ Asked one question at a time	☐ Assessed patient's comprehension of probable illness
☐ Displayed confident manner	☐ Did not use medical jargon	
☐ Showed care and concern	☐ Appropriately used "continuers"	
☐ Was respectful and nonjudgmental	☐ Paraphrased	
☐ Established patient's preferred title	☐ Appropriately used transitions	
☐ Used proper draping	☐ Elicited additional concerns	
☐ Focused on patient	☐ Assessed impact on patient's life	
☐ Did not interrupt patient	☐ Checked for patient understanding	
☐ Maintained appropriate and responsive body language		

Making Decisions	Supporting Emotions
☐ Clearly stated next steps in management	☐ Actively listened and validated patient's expectations
☐ **Counseled** patient	☐ Showed empathy and used appropriate reassurances
☐ Agreed to **mutual plan** of action	☐ Inquired about patient's support system
	☐ Managed the **challenge** (here; patient has difficulty understanding the diagnosis)

History and Physical Examination Checklist

HPI

- ☐ Difficulty swallowing
- ☐ Duration: 1 Month
- ☐ Affects solids
- ☐ Sensation of food stuck in throat
- ☐ No problem with liquids or semi-solids
- ☐ Progressively worse
  - ☐ Initially could compensate by chewing longer
- ☐ Occasional food regurgitation
- ☐ No associated pain
- ☐ No alleviating or aggravating factors
- ☐ Fatigue
- ☐ Bad breath
- ☐ Weight loss
  - ☐ 9 lbs
  - ☐ Unintentional
  - ☐ 1 month or so
- ☐ No nausea
- ☐ No vomiting
- ☐ No diarrhea
- ☐ No blood in stool
- ☐ No fever
- ☐ No chills
- ☐ No SOB

PMH

- ☐ Hx of GERD
- ☐ Treated with antacids
- ☐ No hospitalizations or surgery
- ☐ Meds: aspirin
- ☐ NKDA

Family Hx

- ☐ Father died of lung cancer
- ☐ Mother hx of CAD and HTN

Social Hx

- ☐ Smoked 30 pack yrs
- ☐ Drinks 3-4 glasses of wine/night
  - ☐ CAGE negative
- ☐ No recreational drug use
- ☐ Married with 3 children
- ☐ Works as an accountant

Physical Examination

- ☐ Washed hands prior to examination
- ☐ Inspected oropharynx
- ☐ Inspected thyroid gland
- ☐ Palpated thyroid gland
- ☐ Palpated neck for lymphadenopathy
- ☐ Auscultated abdomen
- ☐ Listened for bowel sounds in 4 quadrants
- ☐ Percussed abdomen in 4 quadrants
- ☐ Palpated abdomen in 4 quadrants

Patient Note

History

CC: 52 yo M c/o difficult swallowing.

HPI: progressive dysphagia to solids, not semisolid foods nor liquids x1 month, described as "food getting stuck in his throat"

No aggrav factors; allev by avoiding meats and breads, no longer allev by chewing longer

Associated Sx / ROS:
+ occ. regurgitation, unintentional 9 lb. wt. loss ×1m, fatigue, halitosis unrelieved with mints

Denies: odynophagia, epigastric or retrosternal pain, bone pain, hoarseness, persistent cough, dyspnea, nausea, vomiting, melena, fever, chills, LAD, abd pain

PMH: GERD. No prior CC, NKDA, hosp, surg, trauma

Allergies: NKDA

Meds: aspirin and Tums as needed

FHx: Father died of lung cancer, mother has CAD and HTN

SHx: cig-30 pack-yrs, ETOH- 3–4 glasses of wine/d, CAGE neg, no drugs.
Married accountant with 3 children

Physical Exam

T 99.1 F, BP 148/78 mm Hg, pulse 74/min, respirations 16/min

GA: appears older than stated age and is thin, but in NAD

HEENT: oropharynx without lesions or tonsillar exudates, good dentition

Neck: no thyromegaly or nodules, no cervical or supraclavicular LAD

Abd: +BS ×4 Q, tympanic to percussion ×4 Q, non-tender, non-distended, no masses or organomegaly

Extr: No CCE

Data Interpretation

DIAGNOSIS 1. ESOPHAGEAL CARCINOMA

History Findings	Physical Exam Findings
Progressive dysphagia to solids	Appears older than stated age and thin
h/o GERD	
30 pack year smoking history	
Daily EtOH use	
9 lb unintentional weight loss	
Sensation of food stuck in throat	
Age	

Diagnosis 2. Esophageal stricture

History Findings	Physical Exam Findings
Dysphagia for solids	Thin-appearing
h/o GERD	
Regurgitation of food	
Unintentional weight loss	

Diagnosis 3. Achalasia

History Findings	Physical Exam Findings
Dysphagia	Thin-appearing
Regurgitation of food	
Unintentional weight loss	

Diagnostic Studies

CXR

Chest CT

Barium esophagram

Esophagogastroduodenoscopy (EGD)

Esophageal manometry

Case Tips and Possible Alternatives

Critical Findings	Case Variations DDX	Important to Communicate
☐ **Progressive dysphagia for solids** ☐ Unintended weight loss ☐ Tobacco and alcohol consumption	☐ Myasthenia gravis (muscle weakness that gets worse w/use, affects extraocular, bulbar or proximal limb muscles, difficulty swallowing, slurred speech, difficulty chewing, bilateral ptosis, progressive)	☐ Care for dysphagia: risks of aspiration pneumonia, choking, nutrition ☐ Tobacco and alcohol cessation ☐ Prep patient for possible bad news (cancer diagnosis)
Note: Recall the impact that a chronic disease will have on a patient's daily life, as well as that of the entire family. It will affect mealtime, hygiene, ambulation, relationships, privacy issues, work, home care. Address these challenges with the patient and family, providing resources to assist.		

CASE 18: SHORTNESS OF BREATH

Doorway Information

Opening Scenario

Mario Hernandez is a 60-year-old man who presents to the ER with shortness of breath.

Vital Signs

T 37 C (98.6 F)

BP 170/95 mm Hg

Pulse 96/min

Respirations 24/min

Oxygen saturation: 90% on room air

Examinee Tasks

1. Obtain a focused history.

2. Perform a relevant physical exam. Do not perform rectal, pelvic, genitourinary, or corneal reflex exam.

3. Discuss your initial diagnostic impression and your workup plan with the patient.

4. After leaving the room, complete your Patient Note on the given form.

Communication and Interpersonal Skills Checklist

Fostering the Relationship	Gathering Information	Providing Information
☐ Knocked	☐ Elicited chief complaint	☐ Summarized significant information
☐ Introduced self	☐ Established timeline of patient's CC	☐ Provided diagnostic impression
☐ Clarified role	☐ Used open-ended question	☐ Justified diagnosis with evidence from encounter
☐ Was properly groomed	☐ Used non-leading questions	☐ Assessed patient's need for additional information
☐ Made eye contact	☐ Used closed-ended questions	☐ Encouraged and answered questions
☐ Maintained appropriate distance	☐ Asked one question at a time	☐ Assessed patient's comprehension of probable illness
☐ Displayed confident manner	☐ Did not use medical jargon	
☐ Showed care and concern	☐ Appropriately used "continuers"	
☐ Was respectful and nonjudgmental	☐ Paraphrased	
☐ Established patient's preferred title	☐ Appropriately used transitions	
☐ Used proper draping	☐ Elicited additional concerns	
☐ Focused on patient	☐ Assessed impact on patient's life	
☐ Did not interrupt patient	☐ Checked for patient understanding	
☐ Maintained appropriate and responsive body language		

Making Decisions	Supporting Emotions
☐ Clearly stated next steps in management	☐ Actively listened and validated patient's expectations
☐ **Counseled** patient	☐ Showed empathy and used appropriate reassurances
☐ Agreed to **mutual plan** of action	☐ Inquired about patient's support system
	☐ Managed the **challenge** (here; patient says, "Doc, I can't breathe.")

History and Physical Examination Checklist

HPI

- ☐ Repeated episodes of shortness of breath
- ☐ Duration: 3 mos
- ☐ Occurs with exertion
- ☐ Progressively worse
  - ☐ Can no longer climb stairs
  - ☐ SOB after walking 1 city block
- ☐ Mild cough
  - ☐ Occasionally productive
  - ☐ Pink tinged, frothy sputum
- ☐ Low grade fever for 2 wks
- ☐ Symptoms worse when he lies down
  - ☐ Wakes up gasping for air when lying flat
  - ☐ Sleeps in a recliner
- ☐ Symptoms improve when sitting upright
- ☐ Swollen legs
- ☐ Weight gain
  - ☐ 10 lbs
  - ☐ Over 1 month
  - ☐ No appetite
- ☐ No chest pain
- ☐ No chills
- ☐ No diaphoresis
- ☐ No wheezing
- ☐ No muscle or joint aches
- ☐ No urinary symptoms
- ☐ No nausea
- ☐ No vomiting or diarrhea

PMH

- ☐ Hx of type 2 diabetes mellitus, HTN, and hyperlipidemia
- ☐ Meds: hydrochlorothiazide, simvastatin, and metformin
- ☐ No hx of surgery
- ☐ NKDA

Family Hx

- ☐ Father died of a heart attack at age 50
- ☐ Brother with hx of HTN and diabetes

Social Hx

- ☐ Smoker: 40 pack yrs
- ☐ Drinks socially
- ☐ Cocaine use for past 4 mos
- ☐ Married with 4 children
- ☐ Retired factory worker

Physical Examination

- ☐ Washed hands prior to examination
- ☐ Performed inspection of chest
- ☐ Performed percussion of lungs bilaterally
- ☐ Palpated for tactile fremitus bilaterally
- ☐ Auscultated lungs
  - ☐ Coughs when asked to breathe deeply or expire fully
  - ☐ Rales 1/3 up from the lung bases
  - ☐ No wheezes
  - ☐ No rhonchi

- ☐ Examined for JVD
  - ☐ JVD halfway to the angle of the jaw
- ☐ Palpated PMI
  - ☐ Laterally displaced PMI
- ☐ Auscultated heart in 4 areas
- ☐ Examined extremities for edema
  - ☐ 2+ pitting edema

Patient Note

History

CC: 60 yo M c/o SOB.

HPI: Presents to the ER with dyspnea on exertion that is progressively worsening for the past 2-3 mos. He has trouble walking up one flight of stairs and becomes very SOB after ambulating less than one city block. He has orthopnea to the point where he now sleeps in a recliner and also reports paroxysmal nocturnal dyspnea. He is a smoker with a 40 pack year history and uses cocaine for the past 4 months.

ROS: + 10 lb wt gain × 1 mo, LE edema, productive cough, pink frothy sputum, intermittent low grade fever ×2wk, anorexia. Denies chest pain, diaphoresis, palpitations, wheezing, weakness, confusion, nausea, nocturia, bloating, abdominal pain, restlessness, dizziness, syncope, fatigue, joint pain, muscle pain, skin changes

PMHx: DM2, HTN, HLD, no surgeries

Medications: simvastatin, metformin, hydrochlorothiazide, NKDA

Family Hx: father died of MI in his 50s, brother has HTN and DM2

Physical Exam

T 98.6 F, BP 170/95 mm Hg, pulse 96/min, respirations 24/min, SaO_2: 90% on room air

General: appears to be in moderate respiratory distress, coughing often when asked to take deep breaths

Chest: symmetrical, normal percussion, normal tactile fremitus, rales 1/3 up from the lung bases, no wheezes or rhonchi

CVS: RRR, normal S1, S2, and +S3 gallop, no murmurs/rubs, PMI is laterally displaced, +JVD halfway to angle of jaw

Extremities: 2+ LE pitting edema

Data Interpretation

DIAGNOSIS 1. CONGESTIVE HEART FAILURE

History Findings	Physical Exam Findings
Progressive DOE	SpO2: 90%, respiratory distress
Orthopnea	Rales on lung exam
Paroxysmal dyspnea	JVD
Leg swelling	S3 gallop
h/o HTN, DM2, HLD	High BP
h/o heavy cigarette smoking	2+ LE pitting edema
FH heart disease	
Cough (pink frothy sputum)	

DIAGNOSIS 2. NON-ISCHEMIC CARDIOMYOPATHY

History Findings	Physical Exam Findings
Progressive DOE	SpO2: 90%, respiratory distress
Orthopnea	Rales on lung exam
Paroxysmal dyspnea	JVD
LE swelling	S3 gallop
h/o fevers	2+ LE pitting edema
h/o cocaine use	

Diagnostic Studies

EKG

Chest x-ray

Echocardiogram

BNP

Urine toxicology

Case Tips and Possible Alternatives

Critical Findings	Case Variations DDX	Important to Communicate
☐ Dyspnea on exertion ☐ **Orthopnea** ☐ **Edema** ☐ H/o cigarette smoking ☐ H/o DM, HTN ☐ **JVD**	☐ Idiopathic pulmonary hypertension (h/o heart murmur, morbid obesity, family history)	☐ Importance of medication compliance ☐ Diet and exercise (lifestyle changes) ☐ Warning signs
Note: Patients are more likely to follow suggestions when they understand their disease and its consequences. If they have more than one chronic ailment, knowing how to manage multiple medications and behaviors can be especially overwhelming. Make sure the patient understands the disease(s), and agree together on an appropriate diet and exercise plan. Instead of saying, "Change your diet. You need to exercise and lose weight," find middle ground so the patient can comply more easily.		

CASE 19: ADULT NOSEBLEED

Doorway Information

Opening Scenario

Kevin Green is a 45-year-old man who presents to your office with chronic nose-bleeds.

Vital Signs

T 36.8 C (98.2 F)

BP 110/80 mm Hg

Pulse 88/min regular

Respirations 18/min

Examinee Tasks

1. Obtain a focused history.

2. Perform a relevant physical exam. Do not perform rectal, pelvic, genitourinary, or corneal reflex exams.

3. Discuss your initial diagnostic impression and your workup plan with the patient.

4. After leaving the room, complete your Patient Note on the given form.

Communication and Interpersonal Skills Checklist

Fostering the Relationship	Gathering Information	Providing Information
☐ Knocked	☐ Elicited chief complaint	☐ Summarized significant information
☐ Introduced self	☐ Established timeline of patient's CC	☐ Provided diagnostic impression
☐ Clarified role	☐ Used open-ended question	☐ Justified diagnosis with evidence from encounter
☐ Was properly groomed	☐ Used non-leading questions	☐ Assessed patient's need for additional information
☐ Made eye contact	☐ Used closed-ended questions	☐ Encouraged and answered questions
☐ Maintained appropriate distance	☐ Asked one question at a time	☐ Assessed patient's comprehension of probable illness
☐ Displayed confident manner	☐ Did not use medical jargon	
☐ Showed care and concern	☐ Appropriately used "continuers"	
☐ Was respectful and nonjudgmental	☐ Paraphrased	
☐ Established patient's preferred title	☐ Appropriately used transitions	
☐ Used proper draping	☐ Elicited additional concerns	
☐ Focused on patient	☐ Assessed impact on patient's life	
☐ Did not interrupt patient	☐ Checked for patient understanding	
☐ Maintained appropriate and responsive body language		

Making Decisions	Supporting Emotions
☐ Clearly stated next steps in management	☐ Actively listened and validated patient's expectations
☐ **Counseled** patient	☐ Showed empathy and used appropriate reassurances
☐ Agreed to **mutual plan** of action	☐ Inquired about patient's support system
	☐ Managed the **challenge** (here; patient asked, "Is it serious?")

History and Physical Examination Checklist

HPI

- ☐ Epistaxis
- ☐ Duration: 3 mos
- ☐ Intermittent
  - ☐ Occurs 1-2 times per week
- ☐ Bleed mostly from left nostril
- ☐ Started after a bad cold
  - ☐ Continued after the cold resolved
- ☐ Quantity of blood
  - ☐ Variable
  - ☐ Severe bleeding twice
- ☐ Self-treatment with tissues up his nose
- ☐ Aggravated by
  - ☐ Sneezing
  - ☐ Blowing his nose

- ☐ Nothing makes it better (self-resolve)
- ☐ No other nasal discharge
- ☐ No recent trauma to nose
- ☐ + bruising easily
- ☐ 10 lbs weight gain
  - ☐ Over 6 mos
  - ☐ Poor diet
    - ☐ Fast food
    - ☐ No vegetables
    - ☐ No fruits
- ☐ Decreased appetite
- ☐ No fever
- ☐ No chills
- ☐ No sore throat
- ☐ No headache
- ☐ No GI bleeding
- ☐ No gingival bleeding
- ☐ Itchy skin
  - ☐ >6 mos

PMH

- ☐ No similar nose prior to these 3 mos
- ☐ No HTN
- ☐ + degenerative joint disease of knee
- ☐ Treated with acetaminophen
  - ☐ 8 tablets per day
- ☐ No hospitalizations or surgery
- ☐ No history of blood transfusions
- ☐ Meds: no prescription meds
- ☐ NKDA

Family Hx

- ☐ No family history of bleeding disorders or blood clots
- ☐ Not been around anyone sick recently
- ☐ Family history of heavy drinking
- ☐ Mother died age late 50s

Social Hx

- ☐ Single
- ☐ Sexually active
- ☐ With women
- ☐ Unsure of HIV status
- ☐ No recreational drug use
- ☐ Previous 2 × 25 pack/yr hx of tobacco
- ☐ Drinks 5 shots of bourbon daily
- ☐ Unemployed
- ☐ Previously a construction worker

Physical Examination

- ☐ Washed hands prior to examination
- ☐ Inspected skin for
  - ☐ Jaundice (+)
  - ☐ Multiple ecchymoses on extremities and trunk (+)
  - ☐ Palmar erythema (−)
  - ☐ Spider angiomata (−)
- ☐ Inspected eye for scleral icterus
  - ☐ Non-injected
  - ☐ (+) scleral icterus
- ☐ Inspected nares
- ☐ Inspected oropharynx
- ☐ Inspected abdomen
- ☐ Auscultated abdomen
  - ☐ +BS in all 4 quadrants

- ☐ Percussed abdomen
- ☐ Palpated abdomen
  - ☐ Soft and non-tender to palpation
- ☐ Assessed abdomen for ascites
  - ☐ No fluid wave
- ☐ Assessed liver and spleen size
  - ☐ No obvious organomegaly
- ☐ Assessed for asterixis
  - ☐ No flapping tremor
  - ☐ AAO × 3
- ☐ Examined extremities for edema
  - ☐ No edema
  - ☐ Thin extremities

Patient Note

History

CC: 45 yo M c/o chronic nosebleeds.

HPI: Left nostril, 1–2 ×/ wk, usually self-resolve, 2 episodes with severe bleeding, onset after URI 3 mos ago; no other nasal discharge.

Aggrav by sneezing or blowing the nose forcefully; allev by pressure from intranasal tissue

ROS: + 10 lb. wt. gain ×6 mos with anorexia, bruises easily, pruritis >6 mos

Denies: hematuria, melena, hematochezia, excessive bleeding/oozing from punctures/incisions, petechiae, purpura, gingival bleeding, breath odor, asterixis, confusion, abd pain, edema, fatigue, nausea, diarrhea, fever, HA, bloating, confusion, somnolence, blurred vision

PMHx: DJD of the knees, no hosp, surg, trauma, HTN, transfusions, NKDA. No epistaxis prior to 3 mos ago.

Meds: Tylenol 8 tabs/d, no Rx meds

SHx: cig-50 pack yrs, ETOH- 5 shots/d, no drugs, single, sexually active w/ women, unemployed construction worker, diet lacks fruits and vegetables

FHx: Mother was a heavy drinker, died in her late 50s.

Physical Exam

BP 110/80 mm Hg, pulse 88/min, T 36.8 C (98.2 F), respirations 18/min

Gen: NAD, slightly disheveled appearance, Skin: jaundiced, multiple ecchymoses on extremities and trunk, no palmar erythema or spider angiomata

HEENT: Eyes: Sclera icteric and non- injected

Nose: L nostril crusted blood w/o active bleeding, R WNL

Oropharynx: poor dentition, but no lesions

Abd: +BS ×4Q, dullness to percussion, soft, NT, no HSM or fluid wave

Extremities: thin, no edema

Neuro: AAO × 3, no asterixis

Data Interpretation

DIAGNOSIS 1. HEPATIC FAILURE

History Findings	Physical Exam Findings
Recurrent epistaxis	Evidence of recent nosebleed
2 episodes of heavy bleeding	Jaundice
Easy bruising, pruritis	Scleral icterus
Weight gain, decreased appetite	Multiple bruises
Excessive acetaminophen use	Dullness to percussion
Heavy drinking history	
Sexually active with multiple women	

DIAGNOSIS 2. NUTRITIONAL DEFICIENCY/VITAMIN C OR K DEFICIENCY

History Findings	Physical Exam Findings
Recurrent epistaxis	Evidence of recent nosebleed
2 episodes of heavy bleeding	Poor dentition
Easy bruising	Multiple bruises
Poor diet	Thin extremities
Heavy drinking	

DIAGNOSIS 3. ITP

History Findings	Physical Exam Findings
Recurrent epistaxis	Evidence of recent nosebleed
2 episodes of heavy bleeding	Multiple bruises
Easy bruising	

Diagnostic Studies

CBC with differential and platelet count

Hepatic function panel (AST, ALT, alk phos, total bilirubin (direct and indirect), total protein, albumin)

PT/INR, PTT, fibrinogen, d-dimer, bleeding time

Acetaminophen level

Vitamin C level

Abdominal U/S

Case Tips and Possible Alternatives

Critical Findings	Case Variations DDX	Important to Communicate
☐ Pruritis >6 months ☐ **Recurrent epistaxis + easy bruising** ☐ Unintended weight gain ☐ Heavy drinking and acetaminophen use ☐ Jaundice	☐ Von Willebrand disease (easy bruising, epistaxis, usually younger age) ☐ Hepatitis C (IV drug user, fatigue, malaise, when advanced: signs of cirrhosis, arthralgias, pruritus)	☐ Education about disease process, alarm signs and symptoms ☐ Nutritional care ☐ Medication management ☐ Alcohol cessation ☐ Safe sex education
Note: A patient who is unemployed and has a chronic disease is at high risk of becoming homeless. It is important to establish level of support the patient has and to provide resources that can help them cope with the burden of their disease.		

CASE 20: ADOLESCENT WEIGHT LOSS

Doorway Information

Opening Scenario

Mr. Wright comes to your clinic to discuss his 14-year-old granddaughter, Amy, who is losing weight.

Vital Signs

N/A

Examinee Tasks

1. Obtain a focused history.

2. You will not be required to perform a physical exam in this case.

3. Discuss your initial diagnostic impression and your workup plan with the patient.

4. After leaving the room, complete your Patient Note on the given form.

Communication and Interpersonal Skills Checklist

Fostering the Relationship	Gathering Information	Providing Information
☐ Knocked	☐ Elicited chief complaint	☐ Summarized significant information
☐ Introduced self	☐ Established timeline of patient's CC	☐ Provided diagnostic impression
☐ Clarified role	☐ Used open-ended question	☐ Justified diagnosis with evidence from encounter
☐ Was properly groomed	☐ Used non-leading questions	☐ Assessed need for additional information
☐ Made eye contact	☐ Used closed-ended questions	☐ Encouraged and answered questions
☐ Maintained appropriate distance	☐ Asked one question at a time	☐ Assessed comprehension of probable illness
☐ Displayed confident manner	☐ Did not use medical jargon	
☐ Showed care and concern	☐ Appropriately used "continuers"	
☐ Was respectful and nonjudgmental	☐ Paraphrased	
☐ Established preferred title	☐ Appropriately used transitions	
☐ Focused on patient	☐ Elicited additional concerns	
☐ Did not interrupt	☐ Assessed impact on patient's life	
☐ Maintained appropriate and responsive body language	☐ Checked for understanding	

Making Decisions	Supporting Emotions
☐ Clearly stated next steps in management	☐ Actively listened and validated expectations
☐ **Counseled** relative	☐ Showed empathy and used appropriate reassurances
☐ Agreed to **mutual plan** of action	☐ Inquired about patient's support system
	☐ Managed the **challenge** (here; grandfather asked, "What can I do?")

History and Physical Examination Checklist

HPI

- ☐ Weight loss
  - ☐ 25 lbs lost
  - ☐ Over 6 mos
  - ☐ Weight 80 lbs
  - ☐ Height 5'3
- ☐ Patient lacks concern about weight loss
  - ☐ Thinks she is overweight
- ☐ Excessive exercise
  - ☐ Hundreds of sit ups each night
  - ☐ Works out with gymnastics team during the week
  - ☐ Works out alone on the weekend
  - ☐ Goal to be on the Olympic team
- ☐ Caloric intake not clear to grandfather
  - ☐ Claims to like food
  - ☐ Pushes about food on her plate at meals
  - ☐ Snacks on carrots and lettuce
- ☐ Menarche at age 12
- ☐ Amenorrhea
  - ☐ >12 mos
- ☐ Heat intolerance
- ☐ Increased sweating
- ☐ Palpitations
  - ☐ Especially after working out
- ☐ Drinks a lot of ice cold water
  - ☐ To cleanse her system
- ☐ No fever
- ☐ No chills
- ☐ No headache
- ☐ No nausea
- ☐ No vomiting
- ☐ No diarrhea
- ☐ No dysuria
- ☐ No easy bruising or bleeding

PMH

- ☐ No history of depression
- ☐ Appears to have recovered from death of mother
- ☐ Emergency appendectomy at age 6
- ☐ Meds: No prescription meds
- ☐ Grandfather discovered laxatives in her room
- ☐ NKDA

Family Hx

- ☐ Mother with history of depression
- ☐ Mother deceased
- ☐ Accident with drunk driver
- ☐ 1 yr ago
- ☐ Grandfather has history of anxiety

Social Hx

- ☐ Lives with grandfather since mother's death
- ☐ Good performance in school
- ☐ Participates in sports
- ☐ Gymnastics
- ☐ Pressure from coach on weight
- ☐ Not sexually active
- ☐ No drug use
- ☐ No smoking
- ☐ No alcohol

Physical Examination

No physical exam

Patient Note

History

CC: 14 yo F who is losing weight.

HPI: 25 lb weight loss over 6 mos. Her grandfather states that she was always thin but now he is concerned. She talks about her love of food but doesn't eat much. She drinks ice cold water excessively "to cleanse her system". Grandfather is not sure about how much she actually eats. She is a gymnast and exercises excessively. She is currently 5 feet 3 inches and 80 lbs, but pt still believes she is overweight. Grandfather found bottles of laxatives in her room.

Associated Sx / ROS: + heat intolerance, diaphoresis, palpitations that increase with exercise, amenorrhea >12mos

Denies: dental erosions, dorsum of hand calluses, thinning hair, lanugo body hair, dry hair, dry skin, cold sensitivity, fatigue, bruising, constipation, vomiting, abd pain, anxiety, syncope, dizziness, peripheral edema, breast atrophy, acrocyanosis, xanthoderma, anxiety, nervousness, tremor, muscle weakness, diarrhea, insomnia.

PMHx: emergency appendectomy at age 6; no h/o depression

Meds: no Rx, + laxative use

Allergies: NKDA

SHx: does well in school; does not drink, smoke, or use illicit drugs. Not sexually active.

FHx: notable for depression in mother, grandfather has anxiety

Physical Examination

N/A

Data Interpretation

DIAGNOSIS 1. ANOREXIA NERVOSA

History Findings	Physical Exam Findings
25 lb weight loss	
Excessive exercising	
Distorted body image	
Amenorrhea	
Laxative use	

DIAGNOSIS 2. HYPERTHYROIDISM

History Findings	Physical Exam Findings
25 lb weight loss	
Amenorrhea	
Palpitations	
Heat intolerance	

Diagnostic Studies

Physical exam

FSH, LH, Prolactin

BUN, creatinine

Electrolytes

Total protein, albumin

EKG

TSH, Free T3 and T4

Thyroid uptake scan

Case Tips and Possible Alternatives

Critical Findings	Case Variations DDX	Important to Communicate
☐ Weight loss ☐ Amenorrhea ☐ Laxative use	☐ Celiac disease (weight loss, weakness, fatigue, abdominal pain, diarrhea, flatulence, amenorrhea, skin changes)	☐ Importance of seeking medical/professional help ☐ Warning signs that merit immediate medical attention
Note: Eating disorders are very complex and require a team of experts to treat underlying causes. It can be difficult for family members to understand that this type of disorder is not a choice. Treatment is highly individual, and needs to be tailored to each patient.		

CASE 21: PEDIATRIC VOMITING AND DIARRHEA

Doorway Information

Opening Scenario

Lilian James is an 18-month-old girl whose mother calls the physician about the child's vomiting and diarrhea for the past 2 days.

Vital Signs

There are no vital signs taken in this case.

Examinee Tasks

1. Obtain a focused history.

2. You will not be required to perform a physical exam in this case.

3. Discuss your initial diagnostic impression and your workup plan with the patient.

4. After leaving the room, complete your Patient Note on the given form.

Communication and Interpersonal Skills Checklist

Fostering the Relationship	Gathering Information	Providing Information
☐ Introduced self ☐ Clarified role ☐ Displayed confident manner ☐ Showed care and concern ☐ Was respectful and nonjudgmental ☐ Established preferred title ☐ Did not interrupt	☐ Elicited chief complaint ☐ Established timeline of patient's CC ☐ Used open-ended question ☐ Used non-leading questions ☐ Used closed-ended questions ☐ Asked one question at a time ☐ Did not use medical jargon ☐ Appropriately used "continuers" ☐ Paraphrased ☐ Appropriately used transitions ☐ Elicited additional concerns ☐ Assessed impact on patient's life ☐ Checked for patient understanding	☐ Summarized significant information ☐ Provided diagnostic impression ☐ Justified diagnosis with evidence from encounter ☐ Assessed need for additional information ☐ Encouraged and answered questions ☐ Assessed comprehension of probable illness

Making Decisions	Supporting Emotions
☐ Clearly stated next steps in management ☐ **Counseled** relative ☐ Agreed to **mutual plan** of action	☐ Actively listened and validated expectations ☐ Showed empathy and used appropriate reassurances ☐ Inquired about patient's support system ☐ Managed the **challenge** (here; mother asked, "Will my baby be okay?")

History and Physical Examination Checklist

HPI

- ☐ Vomiting
  - ☐ 6 episodes
  - ☐ Non bloody
  - ☐ Initially food particles only
  - ☐ Currently bilious
- ☐ Diarrhea
  - ☐ 4 episodes in the past day
  - ☐ Brown stools
  - ☐ Watery
  - ☐ Non bloody
  - ☐ Appears to be in pain with every bowel movement
- ☐ Duration: 2 days
- ☐ Onset
  - ☐ Sudden
  - ☐ 1 day after playdate
  - ☐ No known sick contacts
- ☐ Anorexia
  - ☐ Nothing PO
- ☐ Fever
  - ☐ Low grade fever
  - ☐ Improved with Tylenol
- ☐ No cough
- ☐ No rhinorrhea
- ☐ No shortness of breath
- ☐ No skin rashes or discoloration of the skin.

PMH

- ☐ Recent otitis media
  - ☐ Treated with amoxicillin
  - ☐ 4 weeks ago
- ☐ No hospitalizations
- ☐ No surgery
- ☐ No recent trauma
- ☐ Meds: Tylenol, pediatric multivitamin
- ☐ No other medications
- ☐ NKDA

Ped Hx

- ☐ Full term
- ☐ Delivered by elective cesarean section
- ☐ Adequate prenatal care
- ☐ No complications in neonatal period
- ☐ Mother did not smoke, use drugs or alcohol during pregnancy
- ☐ Breastfed
  - ☐ 8 mos
- ☐ Currently eats
  - ☐ Regular table food
  - ☐ Drinks cow's milk
- ☐ Regular well child visits
  - ☐ Met age appropriate developmental milestones
- ☐ Immunization
  - ☐ Up to date
  - ☐ Except rotavirus

Family Hx

- ☐ Father and mother have no history of acute diarrhea
- ☐ No sick contacts

Social Hx

- ☐ Lives with parents
- ☐ Pet dog

Physical Examination

No physical exam

Patient Note

History

CC: 18 mo F w/ vomiting and diarrhea ×2d

HPI: Sudden onset 1 day after play-date with other toddlers.
Vomited ×6, non-bloody, initially food particles, now bilious.
Diarrhea ×4 in past day, watery with brown non- bloody stools

ROS: + anorexia, poor PO intake, crampy abd pain w/BM, low-grade fever reduced w/ Tylenol
No diaphoresis, oliguria, wt. loss, bloating, lethargy, irritability, cough, rhinorrhea, dyspnea, skin rashes
PMH: Otitis media treated w/ oral ABO 4 wks ago.
No similar CC
No hosp, surg, trauma, sick contacts, NKDA
PedHx: FT born by C/S w/o complications, normal prenatal care, breastfed until 8 mos and now eats regular table food and cow's milk, met age-appropriate developmental milestones, immunizations up to date, except rotavirus vaccine.
Medications: Pediatric MVI, Tylenol PRN fever.
FH: Mother and father are healthy with no chronic illnesses.

Physical Examination

N/A

DIAGNOSIS 1. VIRAL GASTROENTERITIS

History Findings	Physical Exam Findings
Low grade fever	
Non bloody vomitus	
Non-bloody diarrhea	
Acute onset of symptoms	
Incomplete rotavirus vaccinations	
Abdominal pain	

DIAGNOSIS 2. CLOSTRIDIUM DIFFICILE COLITIS

History Findings	Physical Exam Findings
Low-grade fever	
Watery diarrhea	
Recent antibiotic use	
Abdominal pain	
Vomiting	
Anorexia	

Diagnostic Studies

Physical exam

CBC w/ differential

Electrolytes, BUN, creatinine

Stool for *C. difficile* toxin / ELISA for toxin A or B / stool PCR for rotavirus

Stool for fecal leukocytes, ova, and parasites

Blood culture

Fecal lactoferrin

Case Tips and Possible Alternatives

Critical Findings	Case Variations DDX	Important to Communicate
☐ Non-bloody vomitus and diarrhea ☐ Incomplete vaccination schedule ☐ Low grade fever	☐ Bacterial pharyngitis (starting school/daycare, low grade fever, vomiting, h/o sick contacts) ☐ UTI (fever, mild vomiting, abdominal discomfort, fuzziness)	☐ Oral rehydration therapy ☐ Educate about warning signs of severe dehydration ☐ Diet
Note: Nausea and vomiting are common in many disorders, and younger children can have atypical presentations. When seeing pediatric patients, physicians must educate parents/guardians about warning signs of a more serious condition such as dehydration and when to seek immediate medical attention as well as staying calm and collected.		

CASE 22: LACK OF ENERGY

Doorway Information

Opening Scenario

Mr. Dennis Hall is a 55-year-old man who presents with decreased energy for the past 3 yrs.

Vital Signs

T 36.6 C (98.0 F)

BP 130/85 mm Hg

Pulse 90/min

Respirations 12/min

Weight 250 lbs

Height 5 ft 7 in

Examinee Tasks

1. Obtain a focused history.

2. Perform a relevant physical exam. Do not perform rectal, pelvic, genitourinary, or corneal reflex exam.

3. Discuss your initial diagnostic impression and your workup plan with the patient.

4. After leaving the room, complete your Patient Note on the given form.

Communication and Interpersonal Skills Checklist

Fostering the Relationship	Gathering Information	Providing Information
☐ Knocked	☐ Elicited chief complaint	☐ Summarized significant information
☐ Introduced self	☐ Established timeline of patient's CC	☐ Provided diagnostic impression
☐ Clarified role	☐ Used open-ended question	☐ Justified diagnosis with evidence from encounter
☐ Was properly groomed	☐ Used non-leading questions	
☐ Made eye contact	☐ Used closed-ended questions	☐ Assessed patient's need for additional information
☐ Maintained appropriate distance	☐ Asked one question at a time	
☐ Displayed confident manner	☐ Did not use medical jargon	☐ Encouraged and answered questions
☐ Showed care and concern	☐ Appropriately used "continuers"	
☐ Was respectful and nonjudgmental	☐ Paraphrased	☐ Assessed patient's comprehension of probable illness
☐ Established patient's preferred title	☐ Appropriately used transitions	
☐ Used proper draping	☐ Elicited additional concerns	
☐ Focused on patient	☐ Assessed impact on patient's life	
☐ Did not interrupt patient	☐ Checked for patient understanding	
☐ Maintained appropriate and responsive body language		

Making Decisions	Supporting Emotions
☐ Clearly stated next steps in management	☐ Actively listened and validated patient's expectations
☐ **Counseled** patient	☐ Showed empathy and used appropriate reassurances
☐ Agreed to **mutual plan** of action	☐ Inquired about patient's support system
	☐ Managed the **challenge** (here; patient asked, "is it normal to be forgetful at my age?")

History and Physical Examination Checklist	
HPI	**PMH**
☐ Decreased energy	☐ No significant past medical history
☐ Duration: 3 yrs	☐ No hospitalization or surgery
☐ Progressive	☐ Meds: no prescription meds, Colace for constipation
☐ Sleeps 8 hours	☐ NKDA
☐ Does not snore (according to wife)	☐ Has not seen a physician in 2 yrs
☐ Does not need to take naps during the day	**Family Hx**
☐ Weight gain	☐ Maternal uncle with Sjogren syndrome
☐ 5 lbs	☐ No other significant family history
☐ Over 1 year	**Social Hx**
☐ Does not exercise: no energy	☐ Works as an accountant
☐ Tries to eat healthy	☐ No recreational drugs
☐ Forgetfulness	☐ No smoking
☐ Difficulty remembering clients' names	☐ No alcohol
☐ Forgets to complete tasks on time	☐ Married
☐ Assumes it is due to age	☐ Monogamous with wife
☐ Numbness and tingling	
☐ Right hand	
☐ Occasional	
☐ Especially when he wakes up	
☐ Strange feeling in legs	
☐ Change in voice timber	
☐ Recent onset	
☐ Insidious	
☐ Hoarser voice	
☐ Mild cold intolerance/no heat intolerance	
☐ No thinning of hair	
☐ No change in diet	
☐ No swelling of legs	
☐ Constipation: occasionally	
☐ No diarrhea	
☐ No chest pain, no palpitations, no SOB	

Physical Examination	
☐ Washed hands prior to examination	☐ Performed mini mental status exam
☐ Inspected hair	☐ Assessed motor strength bilaterally in hands
☐ Inspected skin	☐ Assessed DTRs
☐ Forearms dry and scaly	☐ Assessed 2 modalities of sensation (light, sharp/dull) bilaterally
☐ Inspected thyroid gland	☐ Sharp sensation decreased
☐ Auscultated neck for thyroid bruits	
☐ Palpated thyroid gland	

Patient Note

History

CC: 55 yo M c/o decreased energy for the past 3 years.

HPI: He complains of progressively worsening fatigue for the past 3 years. He has not seen a physician in over 2 yrs. He works as an accountant and mentions being more forgetful lately. His wife reports that he does not snore at night but that his voice has become hoarser.

ROS: + cold intolerance, occasional paresthesia of R hand, "strange" leg feeling, hoarse voice, 5 lb wt gain ×2y, memory loss, occasional constipation. Denies: dry skin, hair loss, coarse hair, brittle nails, muscle weakness, muscle pain/stiffness, depressed mood, puffy face, sexual dysfunction, pica for ice, dizziness, HA, chest pain, dyspnea, pallor, glossy tongue, angular stomatitis, melena, palpitations, peripheral edema, sleep changes

PMH/SHx: no hospitalizations, no previous surgeries

Meds: Colace, as needed for constipation, no herbal medications, no prescription meds.

Allergies: NKDA

Family Hx: Maternal uncle with Sjogren syndrome

Social Hx: Pt is married, 3 children, monogamous with wife. No h/o EtOH, Smoking, or Rec Drugs

Physical Exam

T 98.0 F; BP 130/85 mm Hg; pulse 90/min; respirations 12/min

Gen: No acute distress. Overweight. Voice sounds hoarse

A&O × 3

Hair not noted to be brittle

Neck: No thyroid bruit; no visible scars or swelling; no thyroid tenderness or enlargement

Neuro: motor strength: 5/5 UE b/l; DTR: 2+; light, dull sensations intact; sharp sensation decreased on palm & front of thumb, index & middle finger of right hand

Skin: forearms dry & scaly

Data Interpretation

DIAGNOSIS 1. HYPOTHYROIDISM

History Findings	Physical Exam Findings
Fatigue	Overweight
Weight gain	Decreased sensation in right hand
Numbness in right hand	Skin dry and scaly
Constipation	
Voice change	
Cold intolerance	
Uncle with history of Sjogren syndrome	
Impaired memory	

DIAGNOSIS 2. IRON DEFICIENCY ANEMIA

History Findings	Physical Exam Findings
Fatigue	Skin dry and scaly
Constipation	
Cold intolerance	
Leg cramps	
Impaired memory	

Diagnostic Studies

Rectal exam, FOB

TSH, T4, FTI

CBC, MCV, RDW

Peripheral smear

Serum FE, TIBC, serum ferritin

Reticulocyte count

Case Tips and Possible Alternatives

Critical Findings	Case Variations DDX	Important to Communicate
☐ Worsening fatigue × 3 years ☐ Weight gain ☐ Impaired memory ☐ Family h/o autoimmune disease	☐ Major depressive disorder (weight changes, fatigue/loss of energy, decreased ability to focus, anhedonia, sleep disturbances) ☐ Addison disease (progressive weakness, poor appetite, nausea, vomiting, diarrhea, skin changes)	☐ Timing and administration of medication ☐ Frequency of follow up ☐ Possible medication interactions
Note: Low thyroid function in men can present as erectile dysfunction and decreased sex drive. Men can have a hard time talking about these issues (as well as decline in mental capacity), so it is up to the physician to remind their male patients about thyroid function.		

CASE 23: CHEST PAIN

Doorway Information

Opening Scenario

Mrs. Simone David, a 53-year-old woman, presents with chest pain for the past 2 hours.

Vital Signs

T 37 C (98.6 F)

BP 150/90 mm Hg

Pulse 86/min

Respirations 20/min

O2 97% on room air

Examinee Tasks

1. Obtain a focused history.

2. Perform a relevant physical exam. Do not perform rectal, pelvic, genitourinary, female breast, or corneal reflex exam.

3. Discuss your initial diagnostic impression and your workup plan with the patient.

4. After leaving the room, complete your Patient Note on the given form.

Communication and Interpersonal Skills Checklist

Fostering the Relationship	Gathering Information	Providing Information
☐ Knocked	☐ Elicited chief complaint	☐ Summarized significant information
☐ Introduced self	☐ Established timeline of patient's CC	☐ Provided diagnostic impression
☐ Clarified role	☐ Used open-ended question	☐ Justified diagnosis with evidence from encounter
☐ Was properly groomed	☐ Used non-leading questions	☐ Assessed patient's need for additional information
☐ Made eye contact	☐ Used closed-ended questions	☐ Encouraged and answered questions
☐ Maintained appropriate distance	☐ Asked one question at a time	☐ Assessed patient's comprehension of probable illness
☐ Displayed confident manner	☐ Did not use medical jargon	
☐ Showed care and concern	☐ Appropriately used "continuers"	
☐ Was respectful and nonjudgmental	☐ Paraphrased	
☐ Established patient's preferred title	☐ Appropriately used transitions	
☐ Used proper draping	☐ Elicited additional concerns	
☐ Focused on patient	☐ Assessed impact on patient's life	
☐ Did not interrupt patient	☐ Checked for patient understanding	
☐ Maintained appropriate and responsive body language		

Making Decisions	Supporting Emotions
☐ Clearly stated next steps in management	☐ Actively listened and validated patient's expectations
☐ **Counseled** patient	☐ Showed empathy and used appropriate reassurances
☐ Agreed to **mutual plan** of action	☐ Inquired about patient's support system
	☐ Managed the **challenge** (here; patient asked, "Should I be worried?")

History and Physical Examination Checklist

HPI

- ☐ Chest pain
- ☐ Duration: 2 hours
- ☐ Acute onset
- ☐ Constant
- ☐ Sharp
- ☐ Not radiating
- ☐ 5/10 severity
- ☐ No change in pain with
  - ☐ Exercise
  - ☐ Feeding
  - ☐ Position
  - ☐ Deep inspiration
- ☐ No shortness of breath
- ☐ No palpitations
- ☐ No diaphoresis
- ☐ No recent travel
- ☐ No trauma
- ☐ No strenuous activity
  - ☐ Sport
  - ☐ Lifting heavy objects
- ☐ OBGYN
  - ☐ LMP
    - ☐ 2 weeks ago
    - ☐ Regular
  - ☐ Para 1
  - ☐ Gravida 1

PMH

- ☐ No similar episodes in the past
- ☐ No recent injuries
- ☐ No history of HTN, heart disease, high cholesterol or diabetes
- ☐ No hospitalization or surgery except child birth
- ☐ LMP 2 wks ago
- ☐ No meds
- ☐ NKDA

Family Hx

- ☐ No family history of diabetes, heart disease, high cholesterol, or hypertension

Social Hx

- ☐ No recreational drugs
- ☐ No smoking
- ☐ Alcohol
  - ☐ 2 glasses of wine/week
- ☐ Married
- ☐ Monogamous
- ☐ No history of STDs

Physical Examination

- ☐ Washed hands prior to examination
- ☐ Inspection of chest & JVP
- ☐ Auscultation of 4 valves of heart and carotids
- ☐ Palpation of chest for tenderness, location of PMI,
  - ☐ Reproducible tenderness of the sternocostal angle
- ☐ Auscultation of lungs
- ☐ Checked carotid & peripheral pulses
- ☐ Examination of extremities for edema and cyanosis

Patient Note

History

CC: 53 yo F c/o chest pain × 2h

HPI: Acute onset, sharp, non-pleuritic, constant, non-radiating, 5/10 in severity,

Not aggrav or allev by food, exercise or position; no strenuous unaccustomed activity

ROS: Denies dyspnea, palpitations, diaphoresis, lightheadedness, syncope, nausea, vomiting, cough, wheezing, frothy sputum, fatigue, malaise, anxiety, indigestion, heartburn, shoulder pain, back pain, abd pain.

PH: No prior episode of CC, Rx, OTC, trauma, surg, NKDA; No h/o DM, HTN, Heart Dx, HLD

OB/GYN: LMP 2 wks ago, reg menses, G1P1; hosp for birth.

SexHx: No h/o STI, monogamous with husband.

SHx: married, (−) tobacco/ illicit drug use, (+) ETOH 2 glasses of wine/wk.

FHx: No similar CC or illnesses (DM, HTN, Heart Dx, HDL)

Physical Examination

T 98.6 F; BP 150/90 mm Hg; pulse 86/min; respirations 20/min O2 97% RA

GA: alert, conscious and coherent; in moderate distress

CV: S1 and S2 normal; RRR; no m, r, g; PMI not displaced; no carotid bruits; no JVD; positive point tenderness on sternocostal angle

Carotids and peripheral pulses palpable and equal b/l 2+

Lung: CTA b/l; no rales, wheezes, rhonchi, or rubs

Extr: no CCE

Data Interpretation

DIAGNOSIS 1: COSTOCHONDRITIS

History Findings	Physical Exam Findings
Chest pain	Normal pulse and O_2 saturation
Acute onset	Point tenderness on sternocostal angle
Constant, non-radiating sharp pain	No palpable edema
Pain is non-pleuritic	
Not associated with SOB or palpitations	
No family h/o DM or heart disease	
No risk factors for heart disease	
No h/o HTN, DM, heart Dx	

DIAGNOSIS 2: ACUTE MYOCARDIAL INFARCTION

History Findings	Physical Exam Findings
Chest pain: sharp, constant	Hypertensive: 150/90 mm Hg
Pain not precipitated by food or deep inspiration	
Acute onset	

Diagnostic Studies

EKG

Chest x-ray

CK-MB, troponin

Case Tips and Possible Alternatives

Critical Findings	Case Variations DDX	Important to Communicate
☐ Acute onset chest pain ☐ No diaphoresis ☐ No family history ☐ No tobacco use or other recreational drugs	☐ Herpes zoster (pre-eruptive phase: can last 10 days, pain, malaise) ☐ Acute pericarditis (pleuritic, sharp, or dull chest pain): pain worse with inspiration or lying flat	☐ Pain management guidelines (medication and possible side effects) ☐ Local heat ☐ Stretching exercises ☐ Modify posture and ergonomic set-up at home/work ☐ Avoid repetitive movements
Note: Chest pain can be the result of many things and can be non-specific. Not every patient with an MI will present with classical signs and symptoms. Record a detailed personal and family history to help establish risk factors.		

CASE 24: KNEE AND GREAT TOE PAIN

Doorway Information

Opening Scenario

Mr. James Hopper is a 58-year-old man who presents with severe pain in his left knee and left great toe for the past 2 days.

Vital Signs

T 37.6 C (99.8 F)

BP 130/80 mm Hg

Pulse 88/min

Respirations 16/min

Examinee Tasks

1. Obtain a focused history.

2. Perform a relevant physical exam. Do not perform rectal, pelvic, genitourinary, female breast, or corneal reflex exam.

3. Discuss your initial diagnostic impression and your workup plan with the patient.

4. After leaving the room, complete your Patient Note on the given form.

Communication and Interpersonal Skills Checklist

Fostering the Relationship	Gathering Information	Providing Information
☐ Knocked	☐ Elicited chief complaint	☐ Summarized significant information
☐ Introduced self	☐ Established timeline of patient's CC	☐ Provided diagnostic impression
☐ Clarified role	☐ Used open-ended question	☐ Justified diagnosis with evidence from encounter
☐ Was properly groomed	☐ Used non-leading questions	☐ Assessed patient's need for additional information
☐ Made eye contact	☐ Used closed-ended questions	☐ Encouraged and answered questions
☐ Maintained appropriate distance	☐ Asked one question at a time	☐ Assessed patient's comprehension of probable illness
☐ Displayed confident manner	☐ Did not use medical jargon	
☐ Showed care and concern	☐ Appropriately used "continuers"	
☐ Was respectful and nonjudgmental	☐ Paraphrased	
☐ Established patient's preferred title	☐ Appropriately used transitions	
☐ Used proper draping	☐ Elicited additional concerns	
☐ Focused on patient	☐ Assessed impact on patient's life	
☐ Did not interrupt patient	☐ Checked for patient understanding	
☐ Maintained appropriate and responsive body language		

Making Decisions	Supporting Emotions
☐ Clearly stated next steps in management	☐ Actively listened and validated patient's expectations
☐ **Counseled** patient	☐ Showed empathy and used appropriate reassurances
☐ Agreed to **mutual plan** of action	☐ Inquired about patient's support system
	☐ Managed the **challenge** (here; patient asked, "Can you give me something for the pain?")

History and Physical Examination Checklist

HPI

- ☐ Left knee pain
- ☐ Left great toe pain
- ☐ Burning sensation
- ☐ Acute onset
    - ☐ Woke him up from sleep
    - ☐ 2 night ago
- ☐ Intensity 9/10
- ☐ Feels sharp
    - ☐ Occasionally dull as well
- ☐ Does not radiate anywhere
- ☐ Increased warmth
- ☐ Swelling of knee and toe
- ☐ No history of trauma
- ☐ Alleviated by ibuprofen
    - ☐ 400 mg
    - ☐ Swelling subsided
    - ☐ Intensity 5/10
- ☐ Exacerbated by pressure from clothing and shoes
- ☐ Previous episode
    - ☐ 4 yrs ago
    - ☐ Also alleviated with ibuprofen
- ☐ No recent injuries to his foot or his knee
- ☐ Started swimming 2-3 × per week to lose weight
- ☐ High protein diet
    - ☐ Red meat most days of the week

PMH

- ☐ Similar episode in past
- ☐ No x-ray taken at the time
- ☐ Did not seek medical attention
- ☐ No history of any chronic condition
- ☐ No surgeries
- ☐ Meds
- ☐ No prescription meds
- ☐ OTC ibuprofen for past 2 days
- ☐ NKDA

Family Hx

- ☐ Non contributory

Social Hx

- ☐ Former smoker
- ☐ 1 pack/day
- ☐ Quit 10 yrs ago
- ☐ No recreational drugs
- ☐ No alcohol
- ☐ Married
- ☐ Works as a photographer
- ☐ Is physically active

Physical Examination

- ☐ Washed hands prior to examination
- ☐ Inspection of lower extremities
- ☐ Palpation of joints in lower extremities
    - ☐ Erythematous and tender to palpation
- ☐ Palpation of peripheral pulses
- ☐ Motor strength of lower extremities
- ☐ Range of motion of lower extremities
    - ☐ Limited painful flexion and extension of affected joints

Patient Note

History

CC: 58 yo M c/o severe pain in his left knee and left great toe for the past 2 days.

HPI: Burning pain which started 2 days ago. Pain is 9/10 in severity, non-radiating, and is exacerbated by any pressure from clothing and shoes. He took ibuprofen, which improved the pain and swelling to 5/10 in intensity. He had similar pain 4 yrs ago for which he took ibuprofen and also improved his pain. At that time, he did not see his PMD and the pain went away within a few days. He denies recent trauma to his left knee and left toe. He does not drink alcohol but does eat red meat most days of the week.

ROS: + swelling and warmth of the knee and toe. Denies: erythema, fever, tophi of soft tissues, flank pain, hematuria, joint stiffness, fatigue, blurred vision, involvement of ankle, wrist, fingers, instep, elbow.

PMH/PSHx: obesity, no major surgeries.

Meds: ibuprofen 1-2 tabs daily for past 2 days

FHx: noncontributory

SH: former smoker, quit 10 yrs ago. No EtOH or recreational drugs. Swims for exercise several times a week

---

Physical Exam

T 99.8 F; BP 130/80 mm Hg; pulse 88/min; respirations 16/min

General: Obese, in moderate distress due to pain of both left great toe and left knee

Extremities: peripheral pulses palpable and equal bilaterally, 2+; no lesions, scars, bruises, discoloration or edema on lower extremities

Musculoskeletal: erythematous, warmth, and tenderness with limited and painful flexion and extension of the left knee and left hallux. No swelling. Other joints of lower extremities bilaterally are nontender and ROM WNL, motor strength 5/5 LE.

Data Interpretation

DIAGNOSIS 1: ACUTE GOUT

History Findings	Physical Exam Findings
Pain in left patellar area and hallux with swelling and warmth	Tender, erythematous, with limited and painful flexion and extension of the left patella and left hallux
Pressure of shoe and clothing exacerbates pain	Warmth
No h/o trauma	Obesity
Pain improved with ibuprofen	
High protein diet (red meat)	
Acute onset	
Previous episode of resolved inflammatory arthritis	
No FH of autoimmune disease	

Diagnosis 2. Calcium Pyrophosphate Deposition (Pseudogout)

History Findings	Physical Exam Findings
Pain in left patellar area and hallux with swelling and warmth	Tender, erythematous, with limited and painful flexion and extension of the left patella and left hallux
Pressure of shoe and clothing exacerbates pain	Warmth
No h/o trauma	
Pain improved with ibuprofen	
Acute onset	
Previous episode of resolved inflammatory arthritis	

Diagnostic Studies

CBC with differential count

ESR, CRP, serum uric acid

Synovial fluid aspiration, fluid analysis with polarizing microscopy, cell count, C&S, Gram stain

X-ray of left knee and left hallux

Case Tips and Possible Alternatives

Critical Findings	Case Variations DDX	Important to Communicate
☐ Severe pain in patellar area and **hallux** ☐ **No h/o trauma or insect bites** ☐ Acute onset ☐ Male	☐ Septic arthritis (acute onset of joint pain, fever, extra-articular symptoms)	☐ Lifestyle changes (weight loss, balanced diet) ☐ Medication compliance
Note: Weight loss is a complex issue to tackle. Patients may find it difficult to make diet modifications and lifestyle changes which include exercise. Make sure the patient sets realistic goals so that success is attainable.		

CASE 25: SEVERE CHEST PAIN

Doorway Information

Opening Scenario

Mr. Dwyane Jackson is a 58-year-old man who presents with chest pain for past 1 hour.

Vital Signs

T 98.6 F (37 C)

BP 128/80 mm Hg

Pulse 110/min

Respirations 22/min

Examinee Tasks

1. Obtain a focused history.

2. Perform a relevant physical exam. Do not perform rectal, pelvic, genitourinary, female breast, or corneal reflex exam.

3. Discuss your initial diagnostic impression and your workup plan with the patient.

4. After leaving the room, complete your Patient Note on the given form.

Communication and Interpersonal Skills Checklist

Fostering the Relationship	Gathering Information	Providing Information
☐ Knocked	☐ Elicited chief complaint	☐ Summarized significant information
☐ Introduced self	☐ Established timeline of patient's CC	☐ Provided diagnostic impression
☐ Clarified role	☐ Used open-ended question	☐ Justified diagnosis with evidence from encounter
☐ Was properly groomed	☐ Used non-leading questions	☐ Assessed patient's need for additional information
☐ Made eye contact	☐ Used closed-ended questions	☐ Encouraged and answered questions
☐ Maintained appropriate distance	☐ Asked one question at a time	☐ Assessed patient's comprehension of probable illness
☐ Displayed confident manner	☐ Did not use medical jargon	
☐ Showed care and concern	☐ Appropriately used "continuers"	
☐ Was respectful and nonjudgmental	☐ Paraphrased	
☐ Established patient's preferred title	☐ Appropriately used transitions	
☐ Used proper draping	☐ Elicited additional concerns	
☐ Focused on patient	☐ Assessed impact on patient's life	
☐ Did not interrupt patient	☐ Checked for patient understanding	
☐ Maintained appropriate and responsive body language		

Making Decisions	Supporting Emotions
☐ Clearly stated next steps in management	☐ Actively listened and validated patient's expectations
☐ **Counseled** patient	☐ Showed empathy and used appropriate reassurances
☐ Agreed to **mutual plan** of action	☐ Inquired about patient's support system
	☐ Managed the **challenge** (here; patient asked, "Am I having a heart attack?")

History and Physical Examination Checklist

HPI

- ☐ Chest pain
  - ☐ Substernal
  - ☐ 7/10 intensity
  - ☐ No radiation
- ☐ Duration 1 hour
- ☐ Started while moving furniture into son's new apartment
- ☐ Prior to pain, patient had a meal at a diner
- ☐ Patient stressed because son is relocating to attend college
- ☐ Pain not relieved by rest
- ☐ SOB
- ☐ No diaphoresis
- ☐ No nausea
- ☐ No recent weight loss or gain
- ☐ Eats a healthy diet

PMH

- ☐ No similar episodes in the past
- ☐ No hospitalizations or surgeries
- ☐ No h/o HTN, DM, HLD
- ☐ Meds: no Rx meds, daily multivitamin, NKDA

Family Hx

- ☐ Father deceased from "heart trouble" at age 67
- ☐ Mother with history of DM and HTN

Social Hx

- ☐ Retired police officer
- ☐ No alcohol
- ☐ No recreational drugs
- ☐ No smoking

Physical Examination

- ☐ Washed hands prior to examination
- ☐ Auscultated the carotids
- ☐ Palpated peripheral pulses bilaterally (radial, DP, PT pulse)
- ☐ Inspected thorax
- ☐ Examined for JVD
- ☐ Palpated chest wall
- ☐ Palpated PMI
- ☐ Auscultated heart in 4 areas
- ☐ Auscultated lungs
- ☐ Examined for cyanosis and edema

Patient Note

History

CC: 58 yo M c/o chest pain ×1h

HPI: Sharp (7/10) sub-sternal without radiation, started while moving furniture after eating, recent stress due to his son relocating for college. No aggrav factors; Rest did not allev his pain, did not try any meds.

ROS: + dyspnea. Denies: pain in back neck jaw shoulders epigastrium, odynophagia, fatigue, dizziness, lightheadedness, diaphoresis, palpitations, anxiety, heartburn, indigestion, nausea, dysphagia, regurgitation, globus, malaise, cough, wheezing, syncope, vomiting.

PMH: No prior episode of CC, Rx, hosp, surg, NKDA; No h/o HTN, DM, HLD

Meds: multivitamins

FH: Father deceased at age 67 of "heart trouble," mother alive with HTN, DM2

SH: Retired police officer, No tobacco, ETOH, drugs; healthy diet

---

Physical Exam

T 98.6 F; BP 128/80 mm Hg; pulse 110/min; respirations 22/min

General: patient appears anxious and in severe distress, holding his chest

Neck: no carotid bruits, no JVD

Cardiac: S1 S2 tachycardic, no M/G/R, no chest wall tenderness, PMI not displaced

Lungs: CTA bilaterally

Extremities: peripheral pulses +2 and equal bilaterally, no discoloration, or edema on upper and lower extremities

---

Data Interpretation

DIAGNOSIS 1. ACUTE MYOCARDIAL INFARCTION

History Findings	Physical Exam Findings
Age >55	Tachycardia
Gender male	Tachypnea
Severe chest pain following strenuous activity	Pt appears to be in severe distress
Substernal location	Cardiac examination without chest wall tenderness
1 hour duration	
Associated SOB	
Not relieved by rest	
Family history of "heart trouble," DM2, and HTN	

DIAGNOSIS 2. ANGINA PECTORIS

History Findings	Physical Exam Findings
Age and gender	Tachycardia
Chest pain following strenuous activity	No tenderness to palpation on examination of chest
Sharp substernal chest pain	Pt in severe distress
Associated SOB	
FH of heart Dx	

DIAGNOSIS 3. ESOPHAGEAL SPASM

History Findings	Physical Exam Findings
Chest pain after eating meal	Normal BP
Stress due to son's relocation	
Not relieved by rest	
No prior episodes of chest pain with exercise	
Severe retrosternal pain	
1 hour duration	

Diagnostic Studies

Troponin, CK-MB

EKG

CXR

Echocardiogram

Case Tips and Possible Alternatives

Critical Findings	Case Variations DDX	Important to Communicate
☐ **Age, gender** ☐ Substernal **chest pain** ☐ 1 hour duration ☐ SOB	☐ Myocarditis (chest pain, palpitations, fever, diaphoresis, h/o flulike symptoms) ☐ Aortic dissection (severe chest pain, syncope, altered mental status, numbness/weakness/ tingling or extremities)	☐ Nothing per mouth (in case of surgical intervention needed) ☐ Stress management (for current situation) ☐ Lifestyle modifications for when patient goes home
Note: Keeping the patient calm and reassuring them is an important step when treating a patient who is having signs and symptoms of an MI.		

CASE 26: CONFUSION AND BLURRY VISION

Doorway Information

Opening Scenario

Ms. Robin Harrison is a 48-year-old woman who presents with confusion and blurry vision for the past 3 hours.

Vital Signs

T 98.6 F (37 C)

BP 230/130 mm Hg

Pulse 88/min

Respirations 22/min

O2 saturation 98% on room air

Examinee Tasks

1. Obtain a focused history.

2. Perform a relevant physical exam. Do not perform rectal, pelvic, genitourinary, female breast, or corneal reflex exam.

3. Discuss your initial diagnostic impression and your workup plan with the patient.

4. After leaving the room, complete your Patient Note on the given form.

Communication and Interpersonal Skills Checklist

Fostering the Relationship	Gathering Information	Providing Information
☐ Knocked	☐ Elicited chief complaint	☐ Summarized significant information
☐ Introduced self	☐ Established timeline of patient's CC	☐ Provided diagnostic impression
☐ Clarified role	☐ Used open-ended question	☐ Justified diagnosis with evidence from encounter
☐ Was properly groomed	☐ Used non-leading questions	☐ Assessed patient's need for additional information
☐ Made eye contact	☐ Used closed-ended questions	☐ Encouraged and answered questions
☐ Maintained appropriate distance	☐ Asked one question at a time	☐ Assessed patient's comprehension of probable illness
☐ Displayed confident manner	☐ Did not use medical jargon	
☐ Showed care and concern	☐ Appropriately used "continuers"	
☐ Was respectful and nonjudgmental	☐ Paraphrased	
☐ Established patient's preferred title	☐ Appropriately used transitions	
☐ Used proper draping	☐ Elicited additional concerns	
☐ Focused on patient	☐ Assessed impact on patient's life	
☐ Did not interrupt patient	☐ Checked for patient understanding	
☐ Maintained appropriate and responsive body language		

Making Decisions	Supporting Emotions
☐ Clearly stated next steps in management	☐ Actively listened and validated patient's expectations
☐ **Counseled** patient	☐ Showed empathy and used appropriate reassurances
☐ Agreed to **mutual plan** of action	☐ Inquired about patient's support system
	☐ Managed the **challenge** (here; patient asked, "Am I having a heart attack?")

History and Physical Examination Checklist

HPI

- ☐ Confusion
- ☐ Blurry vision
- ☐ Duration 3 hour
- ☐ Symptoms worse over past hour
- ☐ Started while she was seated at her desk
- ☐ Presenting symptoms
  - ☐ Headache
  - ☐ Dizziness
  - ☐ Palpitations
  - ☐ Shortness of breath
- ☐ No fever
- ☐ No chills
- ☐ No Nausea
- ☐ No vomiting

PMH

- ☐ No similar episodes in the past
- ☐ HTN, migraine headaches
- ☐ Meds: hydrochlorothiazide, no OTC meds
- ☐ No hospitalizations or surgery, except for childbirths
- ☐ NKDA
- ☐ OBGYN
  - ☐ LMP 2 weeks ago
  - ☐ G2P2
  - ☐ No miscarriages
  - ☐ No contraceptive pills

Family Hx

- ☐ No family history of hypertension, diabetes, or heart disease

Social Hx

- ☐ Alcohol
- ☐ 1-2 glasses of wine/month
- ☐ No recreational drugs
- ☐ No smoking
- ☐ Works as a secretary

Physical Examination

- ☐ Washed hands prior to examination
- ☐ Examined cranial nerves II–XII
- ☐ Performed fundoscopic examination
- ☐ Assessed mental status
- ☐ Examined motor strength
- ☐ Examined sensation
- ☐ Examined deep tendon reflexes
- ☐ Examined cerebellar function
- ☐ Examined gait and tested for Romberg sign
- ☐ Examined for JVD
- ☐ Auscultated carotids
- ☐ Auscultated heart
- ☐ Auscultated lungs
- ☐ Palpated peripheral pulses
- ☐ Examined extremities for edema/clubbing/cyanosis

Patient Note

History

CC: 48 yo F c/o confusion and blurry vision for the past 3 hours.

HPI: She works as a secretary and was sitting at her desk when she suddenly developed these symptoms. They have been progressing over the last hour. She takes hydrochlorothiazide for long-standing HTN, and does not use tobacco products or illicit drugs. She drinks 1–2 glasses of wine a month. Her LMP was 2 weeks ago.

ROS: + HA, dizziness, palpitations, dyspnea. Denies: chest pain, nausea, vomiting, anxiety, seizures, peripheral edema, drowsiness, blurred vision, cough, hemoptysis, hemiparesis, monoparesis, quadriparesis, monocular or binocular vision loss, diplopia, sensory deficits, dysarthria, ataxia, facial droop, vertigo, aphasia, confusion, fatigue, muscle weakness, dysphagia, nystagmus, fever.

PMH/PSHx: No similar episodes in the past. H/o HTN, migraine headaches. No previous surgeries

Meds: hydrochlorothiazide. No over-the-counter medications

Allergies: NKDA

Family history: no HTN, DM2, or heart disease

Physical Examination

VS: T 98.6 F; BP 230/150 mm Hg; pulse 88/min; respirations 16/min

General: Patient in moderate distress, dyspneic

HEENT: No visual field defects, no carotid bruits, no JVD

Fundoscopic exam: sharp disc margins (no papilledema), no hemorrhages or exudates

CV: S1/S2 WNL, RRR, no m, r, or g

Respiratory: CTA bilaterally, no wheezes, crackles, or rhonchi

Extremities: +2 pulses, no cyanosis, clubbing, or edema

Neuro: CN II–XII intact, UE and LE: DTR 2+ bilateral; sharp/dull sensation intact bilaterally; muscle strength 5/5 bilaterally, A&O × 3, RAM intact, normal gait, Romberg negative

---

Data Interpretation

DIAGNOSIS 1. HYPERTENSIVE CRISIS

History Findings	Physical Exam Findings
H/O HTN	BP 230/150 mm Hg
Blurry vision	Patient in moderate distress
Confusion	Dyspnea
Associated headache	No focal neurological findings
Dizziness	
Palpitations	
Dyspnea	

DIAGNOSIS 2. CEREBROVASCULAR ACCIDENT

History Findings	Physical Exam Findings
Blurry vision	BP 230/150 mm Hg
Confusion	Patient in moderate distress
Associated headache	
Dizziness	
H/O HTN	

Diagnostic Studies

Electrolytes

BUN/Cr

U/A

CBC + peripheral blood smear

EKG

Head CT

Case Tips and Possible Alternatives

Critical Findings	Case Variations DDX	Important to Communicate
☐ H/o HTN ☐ Blurry vision ☐ Confusion ☐ Headache ☐ Dyspnea	☐ Aortic dissection (men > women, chest pain, CNS involvement)	☐ Importance of BP control ☐ Medication compliance ☐ Self-monitoring
Note: HTN is particular tricky as patients have a hard time adhering to treatment for a symptomless condition. Educating the patient about consequences of high BP and side effects (transient and otherwise) should be top priority.		

CASE 27: LIFE INSURANCE REQUEST

Doorway Information

Opening Scenario

Mr. John Brown is a 55-year-old man who comes in today for a physical examination.

Vital Signs

Temp 37.0 C (98.6 F)

BP 145/94 mm Hg, right upper limb sitting

Pulse 90/min, regular

Respirations 20/min

Examinee Tasks

1. Obtain a focused history.

2. Perform a relevant physical exam. Do not perform rectal, pelvic, genitourinary, female breast, or corneal reflex exams.

3. Discuss your initial diagnostic impression and diagnostic plan with the patient.

4. After leaving the room, complete the standard patient form that is waiting for you at your desk.

5. Turn in the form that Mr. Brown gives you, but do not write on it.

Communication and Interpersonal Skills Checklist

Fostering the Relationship	Gathering Information	Providing Information
☐ Knocked	☐ Elicited chief complaint	☐ Summarized significant information
☐ Introduced self	☐ Established timeline of patient's CC	☐ Provided diagnostic impression
☐ Clarified role	☐ Used open-ended question	☐ Justified diagnosis with evidence from encounter
☐ Was properly groomed	☐ Used non-leading questions	☐ Assessed patient's need for additional information
☐ Made eye contact	☐ Used closed-ended questions	☐ Encouraged and answered questions
☐ Maintained appropriate distance	☐ Asked one question at a time	☐ Assessed patient's comprehension of probable illness
☐ Displayed confident manner	☐ Did not use medical jargon	
☐ Showed care and concern	☐ Appropriately used "continuers"	
☐ Was respectful and nonjudgmental	☐ Paraphrased	
☐ Established patient's preferred title	☐ Appropriately used transitions	
☐ Used proper draping	☐ Elicited additional concerns	
☐ Focused on patient	☐ Assessed impact on patient's life	
☐ Did not interrupt patient	☐ Checked for patient understanding	
☐ Maintained appropriate and responsive body language		

Making Decisions	Supporting Emotions
☐ Clearly stated next steps in management	☐ Actively listened and validated patient's expectations
☐ **Counseled** patient	☐ Showed empathy and used appropriate reassurances
☐ Agreed to **mutual plan** of action	☐ Inquired about patient's support system
	☐ Managed the **challenge** (here; patient asked, "This isn't a real physical, is it?")

History and Physical Examination Checklist

HPI
- ☐ No fever
- ☐ No chills
- ☐ No cough
- ☐ No SOB or chest pain
- ☐ No changes in bowel habits
- ☐ No blood in the stool
- ☐ No headaches
- ☐ No nausea or vomiting
- ☐ No unintentional weight loss
- ☐ Weight gain
  - ☐ 15 lbs in 6 mos
  - ☐ Patient feels weight gain is due to sedentary job and eating habits
- ☐ Diet
  - ☐ High carbohydrate and fat content
  - ☐ Often feels hungry
- ☐ Increased urination
  - ☐ Increased frequency
  - ☐ Increased volume
  - ☐ No hesitancy
  - ☐ No burning with urination
  - ☐ No blood in urine
  - ☐ No change in the urine stream
  - ☐ Nocturia
  - ☐ Challenging because of job
- ☐ Increased sleep
  - ☐ More than usual
  - ☐ Yet awakes tired and is sleepy during the day
  - ☐ Wife relates that he snores
- ☐ Increased thirst
- ☐ No hoarseness of voice
- ☐ No trouble swallowing
- ☐ Erectile dysfunction

PMH
- ☐ HTN
- ☐ Which patient believes is white coat syndrome
  - ☐ 10 yr history
- ☐ Meds: saw palmetto for increased frequency of urination
- ☐ Cholecystectomy 5 yrs ago
- ☐ NKDA

Family Hx
- ☐ Father and older brother deceased from heart attacks

Social Hx
- ☐ Alcohol
- ☐ 1-2 glasses of wine/week
- ☐ No recreational drugs
- ☐ Past history of smoking tobacco
  - ☐ 1 pack/day
  - ☐ 20 yrs
  - ☐ Quit 1 year ago
- ☐ Works as an air traffic controller
- ☐ Married with no children
- ☐ Not currently sexually active

Physical Examination

- ☐ Washed hands prior to examination
- ☐ Palpated lymph nodes
- ☐ Performed fundoscopic examination
- ☐ Auscultated for carotid bruits
- ☐ Auscultated heart
- ☐ Palpated peripheral pulses
- ☐ Auscultated lungs

- ☐ Inspected abdomen: scar in RUQ
- ☐ Auscultated abdomen
- ☐ Palpated abdomen in 4 quadrants
- ☐ Inspected feet
- ☐ Examined DTRs
- ☐ Checked sensation in extremities: diminished LE stocking pattern
- ☐ Examined extremities for clubbing, cyanosis, and edema

Patient Note

History

CC: 55 yo M comes for a physical examination.

HPI: He has no present complaints.

ROS: + loud snoring, non-restorative sleep, excessive daytime sleepiness, increased somnolence, polyuria, nocturia, frequency, polydipsia, polyphagia, 15 lb wt gain ×6m

Denies: dysuria, hesitancy, hematuria, change in urine stream, blurred vision, LE paresthesias, fatigue, poor wound healing, dyspnea, chest pain, morning HA, dry or sore throat, choking sensation, memory loss, confusion, mood changes, bloody stools, cough, fever, nausea, vomiting, diarrhea, constipation, dysphagia, voice hoarseness, heartburn, peripheral edema.

PMH: HTN × 10y; Hosp/Surg: cholecystectomy

Meds: saw palmetto for frequent urination

No Rx, NKDA

Family Hx: father and older brother died MIs

Sex: Not active w/wife as a result of ED

SH: married and lives with his wife, Smoked 1 PPD × 20 yrs, quit 1 year ago, drinks 1-2 glasses of wine per week, no drugs, works as an air traffic controller, sedentary life, diet high in fat and carbohydrates

---

Physical Exam

T 98.6 F, BP 145/94 mm Hg, right upper limb sitting, pulse 90/min, regular, pulse 20/min

GA: obese individual; not ill appearing

HEENT: no LAD, no carotid bruits

Fundoscopic exam: no hemorrhage, no exudates, no papilledema, no vessel changes

CV: +S1, S2, no m, r, g; RRR

Lungs: CTA bilaterally

Abdomen: cholecystectomy scar, 5 cm in RUQ, + BS in all 4 quadrants, soft, nontender, nondistended, no organomegaly

Ext: no cyanosis or clubbing, edema

Pulses: 2+ throughout

Neuro: diminished sensation in stocking pattern in LE b/l. Feet have no open sores or tenderness. DTRs: 2+ b/l.

Data Interpretation

DIAGNOSIS 1. DIABETES TYPE 2

History Findings	Physical Exam Findings
Weight gain	Obesity
Polyuria	Decreased sensation on neuro exam
Hyperphagia	Hypertension
Polydipsia	
Erectile dysfunction	

DIAGNOSIS 2. OBSTRUCTIVE SLEEP APNEA

History Findings	Physical Exam Findings
Daytime fatigue/tiredness	Obesity
Snoring at night, loud	Hypertension
Increased sleepiness during daytime	
Weight gain	
Nocturia	
Sexual dysfunction	
Male sex	

Diagnostic Studies

Fasting blood glucose

HgA1c

Polysomnography

Case Tips and Possible Alternatives

Critical Findings	Case Variations DDX	Important to Communicate
☐ Weight gain ☐ Polyuria, polydipsia ☐ Erectile dysfunction	☐ Diabetes insipidus (polyuria, polydipsia, fatigue, hair loss)	☐ Importance of glycemic control ☐ Diabetic care (ophthalmology, foot care, renal care) ☐ Diet and exercise
Note: Receiving a new diabetes diagnosis can be overwhelming, as it affects all parts of life and can have severe consequences. Patient education is important and has to be tailored to each patient.		

CASE 28: PRE-EMPLOYMENT PHYSICAL

Doorway Information

Opening Scenario

Mr. Robert Davis is a 40-year-old man who presents for a pre-employment physical examination.

Vital Signs

Temp 38.1 C (100.6 F)

BP 140/90 mm Hg, right upper limb sitting

Pulse 110/min, regular

Respirations 20/min

Examinee Tasks

1. Obtain a focused history.

2. Perform a relevant physical exam. Do not perform rectal, pelvic, genitourinary, female breast, or corneal reflex exams.

3. Discuss your initial diagnostic impression and your workup plan with the patient.

4. After leaving the room, complete your Patient Note on the given form.

Communication and Interpersonal Skills Checklist

Fostering the Relationship	Gathering Information	Providing Information
☐ Knocked	☐ Elicited chief complaint	☐ Summarized significant information
☐ Introduced self	☐ Established timeline of patient's CC	☐ Provided diagnostic impression
☐ Clarified role	☐ Used open-ended question	☐ Justified diagnosis with evidence from encounter
☐ Was properly groomed	☐ Used non-leading questions	☐ Assessed patient's need for additional information
☐ Made eye contact	☐ Used closed-ended questions	☐ Encouraged and answered questions
☐ Maintained appropriate distance	☐ Asked one question at a time	☐ Assessed patient's comprehension of probable illness
☐ Displayed confident manner	☐ Did not use medical jargon	
☐ Showed care and concern	☐ Appropriately used "continuers"	
☐ Was respectful and nonjudgmental	☐ Paraphrased	
☐ Established patient's preferred title	☐ Appropriately used transitions	
☐ Used proper draping	☐ Elicited additional concerns	
☐ Focused on patient	☐ Assessed impact on patient's life	
☐ Did not interrupt patient	☐ Checked for patient understanding	
☐ Maintained appropriate and responsive body language		

Making Decisions	Supporting Emotions
☐ Clearly stated next steps in management	☐ Actively listened and validated patient's expectations
☐ **Counseled** patient	☐ Showed empathy and used appropriate reassurances
☐ Agreed to **mutual plan** of action	☐ Inquired about patient's support system
	☐ Managed the **challenge** (here; ask CAGE questions)

History and Physical Examination Checklist

HPI

- ☐ No cough
- ☐ No SOB
- ☐ No chest pain
- ☐ No palpitations
- ☐ No dysuria
- ☐ No change in bowel habits
- ☐ 2 episodes of nausea and vomiting
  - ☐ No blood
- ☐ No abdominal pain
- ☐ No diarrhea
- ☐ No constipation
- ☐ No numbness/tingling
- ☐ No weight loss
- ☐ No night sweats
- ☐ No joint pain
- ☐ No bruises
- ☐ No difficulty with his hearing or eyesight
- ☐ Feels cold and clammy today
  - ☐ Sometimes feels this way
  - ☐ Goes away in a day or two
  - ☐ Thinks it's a virus
  - ☐ Feels fine otherwise
- ☐ No headache
- ☐ No blurry vision or changes in vision

PMH

- ☐ No history of chronic illness
- ☐ No prior surgeries
- ☐ Hospitalization last month
- ☐ Concussion
- ☐ Required 4 stitches
- ☐ Can't remember what happened
- ☐ Urinated on clothing
- ☐ NKDA
- ☐ No meds

Family Hx

- ☐ Family medical history unknown

Social Hx

- ☐ Not married
- ☐ Lives alone
- ☐ Currently between jobs
- ☐ Alcohol
  - ☐ 6 packs of beer on the weekend
  - ☐ Sometimes during the week as well
  - ☐ Drinks to stop the shakes
  - ☐ Has blackouts
  - ☐ CAGE (3 of 4)
- ☐ Uses recreational drugs
  - ☐ Marijuana
- ☐ Smoker
  - ☐ 1.5 packs/day
  - ☐ 20 yrs
- ☐ Works as a secretary

Physical Examination

- ☐ Washed hands prior to examination
- ☐ Inspected skin
  - ☐ Diaphoretic and tremulous
  - ☐ Spider angioma on the face
  - ☐ Extremities show palmar erythema
  - ☐ Tender lacerations on forehead
- ☐ Inspected oropharynx
  - ☐ Mild tooth decay
- ☐ Assessed mental status
  - ☐ Not oriented to time
  - ☐ His speech is somewhat slow and slurred
  - ☐ He does not make eye contact with you
  - ☐ Short-term memory is poor
  - ☐ He can name 3 objects and does obey commands
  - ☐ He cannot repeat 3 words or spell the word *world* backward

- ☐ Examined cranial nerves II-XII
  - ☐ Extraocular movement appears intact but lateral nystagmus is seen
- ☐ Examined motor strength
  - ☐ Motor strength is normal on left arm and leg, though right arm and leg are noticeably weaker
- ☐ Examined sensation
- ☐ Examined DTRs
- ☐ Assessed cerebellar function
- ☐ Assessed vibratory sense
  - ☐ Gait is ataxic
- ☐ Auscultated heart and lungs
- ☐ Performed fundoscopic exam
- ☐ Abdominal exam

Patient Note

History

CC: 40 yo M presents for a pre-employment physical examination.

HPI/ROS: + nausea and vomiting ×2, feels cold and clammy today, past similar episodes self-resolve in 1–2d.

Denies: hematemesis, HA, gait dysfunction, balance problems, memory loss, change in personality, confusion, blurred vision, weakness, seizures, dizziness, syncope, slurred speech, muscle weakness, dysphagia, incontinence, fatigue, apraxia, diplopia, nystagmus, hallucinations, tremor, anorexia, irritability, fever, insomnia, palpitations, bruises, changes in weight, abdominal pain, changes in bowel habits.

Patient reports that he frequently needs a drink in the morning to prevent "the shakes." He suspects he should feel guilty, and he sometimes wakes up on the floor with loss of urine and isn't sure what happened. He used to be very annoyed by his ex-wife criticizing his drinking, but she left last year.

Meds: none; NKDA

PMH: 1 hosp last month for head trauma, no surgery

SH: lives alone; smoking 30-pack yrs; occ marijuana, binge drinks >6 drinks at a time

CAGE (+) 3 out of 4; drinks frequently to stop shakes

Physical Exam

T 100.62 F, BP 140/90 mm Hg, pulse 110/min, respirations 20/min

GA: unkempt, dirty, diaphoretic, and tremulous. Speech slow and slurred. Poor eye contact

Skin: palmar erythema, spider angioma

HEENT: healing, still-tender laceration to forehead. PERRLA, EOMI, + nystagmus

Oropharynx: mild teeth decay

Fundoscopy: no papilledema

CV: S1 S2 WNL, RRR, no murmur, rub, and gallop, CTAB

Neuro: A&O × 2 to person and place. Poor memory and concentration. Obeys commands and language is intact. CN II- VII intact. Vibration intact in b/l LE

Motor RUE and RLE 3/5. Left side 5/5. Sensation intact. Gait: ataxic; DTR 2+ throughout

Abd: bowel sounds present, nontender, no HSM

Data Interpretation

DIAGNOSIS 1. SUBDURAL HEMATOMA

History Findings	Physical Exam Findings
History of concussion last month	A&O × 2, states year is 1995
Speech somewhat slow, slurred	Poor memory and concentration
"Woke up" on floor	Motor weakness on RUE and RLE 3/5
Incontinence	Laceration to head
2 episodes of nausea and vomiting	+ nystagmus
Risk factor: alcoholism	Gait: ataxic

DIAGNOSIS 2. WERNICKE ENCEPHALOPATHY

History Findings	Physical Exam Findings
Tremors	A&O × 2, states year is 1995
Speech somewhat slow, slurred	Poor memory and concentration
Incontinence	Motor weakness on RUE and RLE 3/5
Binge drinking >6 drinks at a time	Palmar erythema/spider angiomata
CAGE 3/4 positive	Nystagmus
2 episodes of nausea and vomiting	Gait: ataxic
	Tachycardia

DIAGNOSIS 3. ALCOHOL WITHDRAWAL SYNDROME

History Findings	Physical Exam Findings
Tremors	Palmar erythema/spider angiomata
Speech somewhat slow, slurred	A&O × 2, states year is 1995
History of concussion last month	Poor memory and concentration
Incontinence	Tachycardia
Woke up on floor	Fever
Binge drinking >6 drinks at a time	
CAGE 3/4 positive	
2 episodes of nausea and vomiting	

Diagnostic Studies

PT/PPT/INR, platelet count

CBC w/diff, glucose, ammonia level

Serum EtOH levels

CT/MRI of head

Total bilirubin, AST, ALT, GGT

EEG

Vit B1 level

Case Tips and Possible Alternatives

Critical Findings	Case Variations DDX	Important to Communicate
☐ Recent h/o concussion ☐ Slurred, slow speech ☐ Incontinence ☐ Alcoholism	☐ Meningitis (nausea, vomiting, irritability, delirium, fever, neck stiffness)	☐ Alcohol cessation ☐ Smoking cessation ☐ Finding support and counseling
Note: Alcohol use is the 4th leading cause of preventable deaths in the United States. Physicians must emphasize not only the effects it has on health but also the effects it can have on one's occupation, family, and relationships.		

CASE 29: MEDICATION REFILL

Doorway Information

Opening Scenario

Mr. Paul Thomas is a 49-year-old man who calls to request a refill of his medication.

Vital Signs

No vital signs are given in this case.

Examinee Tasks

1. Obtain a focused history.

2. Discuss your initial diagnostic impression and your workup plan with the patient.

3. After ending the call, complete your Patient Note on the given form.

Communication and Interpersonal Skills Checklist

Fostering the Relationship	Gathering Information	Providing Information
☐ Introduced self	☐ Elicited chief complaint	☐ Summarized significant information
☐ Clarified role	☐ Established timeline of patient's CC	☐ Provided diagnostic impression
☐ Maintained appropriate distance	☐ Used open-ended question	☐ Justified diagnosis with evidence from encounter
☐ Displayed confident manner	☐ Used non-leading questions	☐ Assessed patient's need for additional information
☐ Showed care and concern	☐ Used closed-ended questions	☐ Encouraged and answered questions
☐ Was respectful and nonjudgmental	☐ Asked one question at a time	☐ Assessed patient's comprehension of probable illness
☐ Established preferred title	☐ Did not use medical jargon	
☐ Did not interrupt	☐ Appropriately used "continuers"	
	☐ Paraphrased	
	☐ Appropriately used transitions	
	☐ Elicited additional concerns	
	☐ Assessed impact on patient's life	
	☐ Checked for understanding	

Making Decisions	Supporting Emotions
☐ Clearly stated next steps in management	☐ Actively listened and validated patient's expectations
☐ **Counseled** patient	☐ Showed empathy and used appropriate reassurances
☐ Agreed to **mutual plan** of action	☐ Inquired about patient's support system
	☐ Managed the **challenge** (here; patient asked, "are these questions really necessary?")

History and Physical Examination Checklist

HPI

- ☐ Checks BP regularly
  - ☐ Systolic
    - ☐ 120-130 mmHg
  - ☐ Diastolic
    - ☐ 70-84 mmHg
- ☐ No fever
- ☐ No chills
- ☐ No headaches
- ☐ No changes in vision
- ☐ No chest pain
- ☐ Mild SOB
  - ☐ When climbing 2 flights of stairs
- ☐ Ankle edema
- ☐ Dry cough
- ☐ Symptoms in the past 2 mos
- ☐ Weight gain
  - ☐ 15 lbs over 2 mos
  - ☐ No change in appetite
- ☐ Recently needs more pillows to sleep

PMH

- ☐ No hospitalization, no surgeries
- ☐ No history of diabetes, cancer, or heart disease
- ☐ HTN × 10 yrs
- ☐ Medications: lisinopril 10 mg PO daily
  - ☐ Compliant with medication
  - ☐ On drug for 4 yrs
  - ☐ Last physician visit 14 mos ago
- ☐ NKDA

Family Hx

- ☐ No family history of hypertension, diabetes, or heart disease

Social Hx

- ☐ Lives at home with wife of 25 yrs
- ☐ Works as an accountant
- ☐ No alcohol
  - ☐ No recreational drugs
- ☐ No smoking

Physical Examination

No physical exam

Patient Note

History

CC: 49 yo M calls to request a refill of his medication.

HPI: Well controlled HTN ×10y, BP 120-130/70-84, Takes Lisinopril, Last MD visit 14 mos ago.

ROS: + In past 2 mos DOE, dry cough, 15 lb wt gain, LE edema, 1 additional pillow orthopnea. Denies: chest pain, dyspnea at rest, diaphoresis, palpitations, PND, nocturia, fatigue, HA, blurred vision, oliguria, nausea, vomiting, confusion, restlessness, muscle weakness, abdominal pain, fever, dizziness, diarrhea, rash, arthralgia, alopecia, mood changes, hypersomnia, rhinorrhea, sexual dysfunction, sore throat.

PMH: HTN; no DM or Heart Dx, hosp, surg.

Meds: Lisinopril 10mg PO daily, no OTC

SH: Married, accountant, no change in stress level. No tobacco, ETOH, drugs.

FH: No HTN, DM, Heart Dx.

Physical Exam

N/A

Data Interpretation

DIAGNOSIS 1. CONGESTIVE HEART FAILURE

History Findings	Physical Exam Findings
History of HTN	
15-lb weight gain, no change in appetite	
Dyspnea on exertion	
2-pillow orthopnea	
LE edema	
Nonproductive cough	

DIAGNOSIS 2. RENAL INSUFFICIENCY

History Findings	Physical Exam Findings
History of HTN	
LE edema	
Dyspnea on exertion	
15-lb weight gain, no change in appetite	
Use of lisinopril	

DIAGNOSIS 3. DRUG-INDUCED COUGH

History Findings	Physical Exam Findings
Use of lisinopril	
Non-productive cough	
No fever or chills	

Diagnostic Studies

Physical examination

CBC w/ diff

Serum electrolytes, BUN/creatinine, albumin, BNP

Total cholesterol, HDL, LDL, triglycerides

UA, urine electrolytes

EKG

Chest x-ray

Echocardiogram

Case Tips and Possible Alternatives

Critical Findings	Case Variations DDX	Important to Communicate
☐ Long standing HTN ☐ DOE ☐ Orthopnea ☐ LE edema ☐ Cough	☐ ＿＿＿	☐ Importance of medical follow-up
Note: Patients who come for medication refill require a thorough examination. Sometimes the changes can be subtle (as in this case) and the patient might not give it the importance it merits. Changes in weight, quality of sleep, etc. can be slow and insidious.		

CASE 30: BREAKING BAD NEWS

Doorway Information

Opening Scenario

Mr. Paul Harris is a 68-year-old man who had a prostate biopsy last week and is here to receive the pathology results. The results show he has adenocarcinoma of the prostate, and your task is to inform him.

Vital Signs

No vital signs are given in this case.

Examinee Tasks

1. Tell the patient he has prostate cancer.

2. There is no physical exam in this case.

3. Elicit original chief complaint and obtain HPI based on that complaint.

4. After leaving the room, complete your Patient Note on the given form.

Communication and Interpersonal Skills Checklist

Fostering the Relationship	Gathering Information	Providing Information
☐ Knocked	☐ Elicited chief complaint	☐ Summarized significant information
☐ Introduced self	☐ Established timeline of patient's CC	☐ Provided diagnostic impression
☐ Clarified role	☐ Used open-ended question	☐ Justified diagnosis with evidence from encounter
☐ Was properly groomed	☐ Used non-leading questions	
☐ Made eye contact	☐ Used closed-ended questions	☐ Assessed patient's need for additional information
☐ Maintained appropriate distance	☐ Asked one question at a time	
☐ Displayed confident manner	☐ Did not use medical jargon	☐ Encouraged and answered questions
☐ Showed care and concern	☐ Appropriately used "continuers"	
☐ Was respectful and nonjudgmental	☐ Paraphrased	☐ Assessed patient's comprehension of probable illness
☐ Established patient's preferred title	☐ Appropriately used transitions	
☐ Focused on patient	☐ Elicited additional concerns	
☐ Did not interrupt patient	☐ Assessed impact on patient's life	
☐ Maintained appropriate and responsive body language	☐ Checked for patient understanding	

Making Decisions	Supporting Emotions
☐ Clearly stated next steps in management	☐ Actively listened and validated patient's expectations
☐ **Counseled** patient	☐ Showed empathy and used appropriate reassurances
☐ Agreed to **mutual plan** of action	☐ Inquired about patient's support system
	☐ Managed the **challenge** (here; patient asked, "what are my options?")

History and Physical Examination Checklist	
HPI	**PMH**
☐ Positive results of recent prostate biopsy	☐ Hospitalized for tonsillectomy at age 13
☐ Difficulty urinating	☐ Meds: daily multivitamin, no Rx meds
☐ Increased urgency	☐ NKDA
☐ Increased frequency	**Family Hx**
☐ Hesitancy initiating urination	☐ Both parents deceased due to old age
☐ Weak urinary stream	☐ Father at age 89
☐ No change in urine color	☐ Mother at age 93
☐ Nocturia	**Social Hx**
☐ Duration 3 mos	☐ He is a retired attorney
☐ Elevated PSA prompted biopsy	☐ Alcohol
☐ No fever	☐ 1-2 glasses of wine/week
☐ No chills	☐ No recreational drugs
☐ No fatigue	☐ Except some marijuana in college
☐ No polydipsia	☐ No smoking
☐ No dysuria	☐ Sexually active with his wife only
☐ No impotence	☐ Has never been diagnosed with any sexually transmitted disease
☐ No change in his bowel habits	
☐ No change to appetite or weight	
☐ No body aches	
☐ Eats a balanced diet	

Physical Examination
No physical exam

Patient Note

History

CC: 68 yo M who had a prostate biopsy last week and is here to receive the pathology results.

HPI: Biopsy prompted by elevated PSA.

ROS: + 3 mo h/o urgency, frequency, hesitancy, difficulty initiating and maintaining urinary stream, nocturia. Denies: fatigue, wt loss, anorexia, hematuria, dysuria, LE edema, pain in low back hips pelvis thighs, rectal pain/pressure, painful ejaculations, diminished ejaculations, sexual dysfunction, urinary retention, fever, change in urine color, change in bowel habits.

PMH/PSH: tonsillectomy at age 13, otherwise no significant PMH

Meds: multivitamins, no Rx meds

Allergies: NKDA

FHx: father and mother deceased due to old age, at age 89 and 93, respectively

SH: retired attorney, married, sexually active with wife. Social alcohol use, 1-2 glasses of wine/week; no tobacco use, occasional marijuana use in college, eats a balanced diet

Physical Exam

N/A

Data Interpretation

DIAGNOSIS 1. ADENOCARCINOMA OF THE PROSTATE

History Findings	Physical Exam Findings
Urinary urgency	
Urinary frequency	
Urinary hesitancy	
Weak urine stream	
Nocturia	
Elevated PSA	
Positive biopsy results	

Diagnostic Studies

Physical exam

Bone scan

CT scan of abd and pelvis

Case Tips and Possible Alternatives

Critical Findings	Case Variations DDX	Important to Communicate
☐ Urinary urgency, frequency, hesitancy ☐ Weak urine stream	☐ –	☐ Support the patient ☐ Next steps if patient is open to that
Note: Delivering bad news is a very complex task. Reviewing the SPIKES protocol can be helpful both to the patient as well as to the physician.		

CASE 31: WEAKNESS

Doorway Information

Opening Scenario

Kristen Shore is a 24-year-old woman who comes to the office complaining of weakness for 2 months.

Vital Signs

T 37.2 C (98.9 F)

BP 115/77 mm Hg

Pulse 67/min

Respirations 16/min

Examinee Tasks

1. Obtain a focused history.

2. Perform a relevant physical exam. Do not perform rectal, pelvic, genitourinary, female breast, or corneal reflex exam.

3. Discuss your initial diagnostic impression and your workup plan with the patient.

4. After leaving the room, complete your Patient Note.

Communication and Interpersonal Skills Checklist

Fostering the Relationship	Gathering Information	Providing Information
☐ Knocked	☐ Elicited chief complaint	☐ Summarized significant information
☐ Introduced self	☐ Established timeline of patient's CC	☐ Provided diagnostic impression
☐ Clarified role	☐ Used open-ended question	☐ Justified diagnosis with evidence from encounter
☐ Was properly groomed	☐ Used non-leading questions	☐ Assessed patient's need for additional information
☐ Made eye contact	☐ Used closed-ended questions	☐ Encouraged and answered questions
☐ Maintained appropriate distance	☐ Asked one question at a time	☐ Assessed patient's comprehension of probable illness
☐ Displayed confident manner	☐ Did not use medical jargon	
☐ Showed care and concern	☐ Appropriately used "continuers"	
☐ Was respectful and nonjudgmental	☐ Paraphrased	
☐ Established patient's preferred title	☐ Appropriately used transitions	
☐ Used proper draping	☐ Elicited additional concerns	
☐ Focused on patient	☐ Assessed impact on patient's life	
☐ Did not interrupt patient	☐ Checked for patient understanding	
☐ Maintained appropriate and responsive body language		

Making Decisions	Supporting Emotions
☐ Clearly stated next steps in management	☐ Actively listened and validated patient's expectations
☐ **Counseled** patient	☐ Showed empathy and used appropriate reassurances
☐ Agreed to **mutual plan** of action	☐ Inquired about patient's support system
	☐ Managed the **challenge** (here; patient is irritable)

History and Physical Examination Checklist

HPI

☐ Fatigue and weakness
  ☐ Duration: 2 months
  ☐ Progressive
☐ Blurry vision
☐ Double vision
  ☐ Episodic
  ☐ Worse when going up and down stairs
☐ Slurred speech
  ☐ After a prolonged talk
☐ Jaw weakness
  ☐ Difficulty chewing food
  ☐ No difficulty swallowing
☐ Symptoms improve with rest
☐ Worse toward end of the day
☐ No headache
☐ No fever
☐ No chills
☐ No rash
☐ No joint pain
☐ No seizures
☐ No heat/cold intolerance
☐ No SOB
☐ No palpitations
☐ Diarrhea
  ☐ Episode prior to current symptoms
☐ No constipation
☐ No urinary changes
☐ No night sweats
☐ No weight change

PMH

☐ Recent infectious diarrhea
  ☐ 2 months ago
☐ No hospitalization or surgery
☐ Meds: oral contraceptives, no OTC
☐ NKDA
☐ LMP 2 weeks ago
☐ P0 G0

Family Hx

☐ Mother has hypothyroidism
☐ No other significant family history

Social Hx

☐ Mechanical engineering graduate student
☐ No recreational drugs
☐ No smoking
☐ No alcohol
☐ Single
  ☐ Not sexually active

Physical Examination

☐ Washed hands prior to examination
☐ Examined oropharynx
☐ Assessed mental status
☐ Examined cranial nerves II–XII
  ☐ Mild bilateral ptosis which is worsened by prolonged upward gaze
☐ Examined motor strength
☐ Examined sensation
☐ Examined DTRs
☐ Assessed gait
☐ Assessed Romberg
☐ Assessed plantar reflex
☐ Auscultated lungs

Patient Note

History

CC: 24 yo F c/o weakness ×2m

HPI: Progressive, significantly during past week, with episodic diplopia, blurred vision, jaw weakness and slurred speech. Aggrav: diplopia by walking up and down the stairs, dysarthria by prolonged talking, jaw by mastication and all by full day exertion. Allev by rest.

ROS: + As above and fatigue.

Denies: ptosis, dysphagia, neck or extremity weakness, unsteady gait, dyspnea, diaphoresis, anhidrosis, extremity paresthesias or numbness, facial droop, urinary retention, shoulder/ back/hip pain, nausea, vomiting, dry mouth, dry eyes, malaise, dizziness, abd pain, bloating, constipation, current diarrhea, heat or cold intolerance, fever, rash, joint pain, wt change

PMH: Infectious diarrhea 2 mos ago, no prior episode of CC. No hosp, surg, h/o thyroid problems.

Meds: OCP, no OTC. NKDA

OBGYN: G0P0, LMP 2 wks ago

SHx: does not drink, smoke, or use drugs; currently a graduate student; single.

FHx: mother has hypothyroidism.

Physical Examination

T 37.2 C (98.9 F); BP 115/77 mm Hg; pulse 67/min; respirations 16/min

GA: NAD

Oropharynx: no lesions

Lungs: CTA bilaterally, no wheezes or crackles

Neuro: AAO × 3, PERRLA, mild bilateral ptosis which is worsened by prolonged upward gaze. CN II–XII intact, motor 5/5 UE/LE sensation intact to sharp/dull; plantar reflexes WNL. DTRs 2+ and symmetric, no intention tremor or gait abnormalities, Romberg negative

---

Data Interpretation

DIAGNOSIS 1. MYASTHENIA GRAVIS

History Findings	Physical Exam Findings
Progressive fatigue	Ptosis that worsens with prolonged upward gaze
Blurry vision/diplopia	Normal plantar reflex
Jaw weakness and weakness with chewing	
Slurred speech	
Female in third decade	
FH hypothyroidism	
Weakness increased w/ exertion and alleviated by rest	
Worsens as day progresses	

DIAGNOSIS 2. GUILLAIN-BARRE SYNDROME

History Findings	Physical Exam Findings
Progressive fatigue	Ptosis
Blurry vision/diplopia	Normal plantar reflex
Symptoms preceded by diarrheal illness	
Slurred speech	

DIAGNOSIS 3. BOTULISM

History Findings	Physical Exam Findings
Progressive fatigue	Ptosis
Blurry vision/diplopia	Normal plantar reflex
Jaw weakness and weakness with chewing	
Slurred speech	

Diagnostic Studies

Acetylcholine receptor antibodies

Muscle specific tyrosine kinase antibodies, anti-striated muscle antibodies (anti-SM)

Botulinum toxin blood test

FVC, negative inspiratory force (NIF)

Tensilon test

EMG, NCS

Chest x-ray

Case Tips and Possible Alternatives

Critical Findings	Case Variations DDX	Important to Communicate
☐ Progressive fatigue ☐ Diplopia ☐ Slurred speech ☐ Weakness gets worse as day progresses ☐ Alleviated by rest	☐ Lambert-Eaton myasthenic syndrome (usually age >60, slow progression, proximal muscle weakness)	☐ Wellness strategies related to MG ☐ Conserving energy, staying cool ☐ Special diet modifications
Note: Patients who live with conditions that affect many aspects of their life might need help understanding their rights under the Americans with Disability Act (ADA). Physicians should help patients navigate the resources available to better understand the changes that will be needed at home and at work.		

PART VI

Appendix

Common Medical Abbreviations

Use abbreviations sparingly. For clarity, it is always better to spell out the acronym or abbreviation.

4Q	4 quadrants
yo or y/o	year old
m	male
f	female
b	black
w	white
L	left
R	right
hx	history
h/o	history of
c/o	complaining/complaints of
c	with
NL	normal limits
s	without
WNL	within normal limits
Ø	without or no
+	positive
–	negative

A&0x3	alert & oriented to person, place, and time
AA	Alcoholics Anonymous
AAA	abdominal aortic aneurysm
abd	abdomen

ABG	arterial blood gas
ACTH	adrenocorticotropic hormone
ADH	antidiuretic hormone
AFB	acid-fast bacilli
afib	atrial fibrillation
AIDS	acquired immune deficiency syndrome
Alb	albumin
Alk phos	alkaline phosphatase
ALS	amyotrophic lateral sclerosis
ant	anterior
A&P	auscultation and percussion
ARDS	acute respiratory distress syndrome
AV	arteriovenous
AP	anteroposterior
approx	approximately
ASA	aspirin

b/l	bilateral
BID	twice a day
BM	bowel movement
BP	blood pressure

BPH	benign prostatic hypertrophy
BUN	blood urea nitrogen
Bx	biopsy

Ca	calcium
CA	cancer
CABG	coronary artery bypass grafting
CAD	coronary artery disease
cath	catheterization
CBC	complete blood count
cc	chief complaint
CCU	cardiac care unit
CF	cystic fibrosis
Chemo	chemotherapy
CHF	congestive heart failure
chol	cholesterol
cig	cigarettes
Cl	chloride
CMV	cytomegalovirus
CN	cranial nerve
CNS	central nervous system
c/o	complains of
COPD	chronic obstructive pulmonary disease
CPK	creatine phosphokinase
CPR	cardiopulmonary resuscitation
Cr	creatinine
C&S, C/S	culture and sensitivity
CSF	cerebrospinal fluid
CT	computed tomography
CTA	clear to auscultation

CVA	cerebrovascular accident
CVP	central venous pressure
Cx	cervix
CXR	chest x-ray

D&C	dilatation and curettage
d/c	discontinue
DI	diabetes insipidus
DM	diabetes mellitus
DTR	deep tendon reflexes
DVT	deep vein thrombosis
dx	diagnosis

ECG/EKG	electrocardiogram
EEG	electroencephalogram
ED	emergency department
EGD	esophagogastroduodenoscopy
EMG	electromyogram
EMT	emergency medical technician
ENT	ears, nose, and throat
EOMI	extraocular muscles intact
ER	emergency room
ERCP	endoscopic retrograde cholangiopancreatography
ESR	erythrocyte sedimentation rate
EtOH	alcohol
ext	extremities

FBS	fasting blood sugar
Fe	iron

FSH	follicle stimulating hormone
FH	family history
FUO	fever of unknown origin
Fx	fracture

GA	general appearance
GERD	gastroesophageal reflux disorder
GI	gastrointestinal
Glu	glucose
GSW	gunshot wound
GTT	glucose tolerance test
GU	genitourinary

HA	headache
Hct	hematocrit
HEENT	head, eyes, ears, nose, and throat
Hgb	hemoglobin
HIV	human immunodeficiency virus
HRT	hormone replacement therapy
HPI	history of present illness
H. pylori	*Helicobacter pylori*
HR	heart rate
HSM	hepatosplenomegaly
HTN	hypertension

IBS	irritable bowel syndrome
ICU	intensive care unit
IDDM	insulin-dependent diabetes mellitus
IM	intramuscularly

INR	international ratio
IUD	intrauterine device
IV	intravenously

JVD	jugular venous distension
JVP	jugular venous pressure

K	potassium
KUB	kidney, ureter, and bladder

LAD	lymphadenopathy or left anterior descending
LDH	lactate dehydrogenase
LE	lower extremity
LH	luteinizing hormone
LLL	left lower lobe
LLQ	left lower quadrant
LMP	last menstrual period
loc	loss of consciousness
LP	lumbar puncture
LUL	left upper lobe
LUQ	left upper quadrant

M, R, G	murmurs, rubs, or gallops
meds	medications
mets	metastases
MI	myocardial infarction
MRI	magnetic resonance imaging
MS	multiple sclerosis
MVA	motor vehicle accident
MVP	mitral valve prolapse

Na	sodium
NAD	no apparent distress
NC/AT	normocephalic atraumatic
neg	negative
neuro	neurologic
NIDDM	non–insulin-dependent diabetes mellitus
NKA	no known allergies
NKDA	no known drug allergy
NPH	normal pressure hydrocephalus
NSR	normal sinus rhythm
N/V	nausea and vomiting

occ	occasional
OCP	oral contraceptives
OD	right eye
OS	left eye
OTC	over-the-counter

PA	posteroanterior
PCP	primary care provider
PCP	*pneumocystis carinii* pneumonia
PE	physical examination
PE	pulmonary embolus
PERRLA	pupils are equal, round, and reactive to light and accommodation
PET scan	positron emission tomography
PFTs	pulmonary function tests
PID	pelvic inflammatory disease

PMI	point of maximum impulse
po	orally
pos	positive
PPD	packs per day
PPD	purified protein derivative
PRN	as needed
PSA	prostatic specific antigen
PT	prothrombin time
PTT	partial prothrombin time
PUD	peptic ulcer disease
PVD	peripheral vascular disease

r/o	rule out
RA	rheumatoid arthritis
RBC	red blood cells
RLL	right lower lobe
RLQ	right lower quadrant
RMG	rubs, murmurs, or gallops
ROM	range of motion
RR	respiratory rate
RRR	regular rate and rhythm
RUL	right upper lobe
RUQ	right upper quadrant
Rx	prescription

SH	social history
SLE	systemic lupus erythematosus
SLR	straight leg raising
sob	shortness of breath
SQ	subcutaneous

Staph	staphylococcus
STD	sexually transmitted disease
Strep	streptococcus

T	temperature
TB	tuberculosis
TIA	transient ischemic attack
TSH	thyroid stimulating hormone
TURP	transurethral prostatectomy
TVF	tactile vocal fremitus

U/A	urinalysis
UE	upper extremity
UGI	upper gastrointestinal
URI	upper respiratory tract infection
U/S	ultrasound
UTI	urinary tract infection

vag	vaginal
VCUG	voiding cystourethrogram
VDRL	Venereal Disease Research Laboratory
vs	vital signs

w/	with
WBC	white blood cells
wks	weeks
WNL	within normal limits
wt	weight

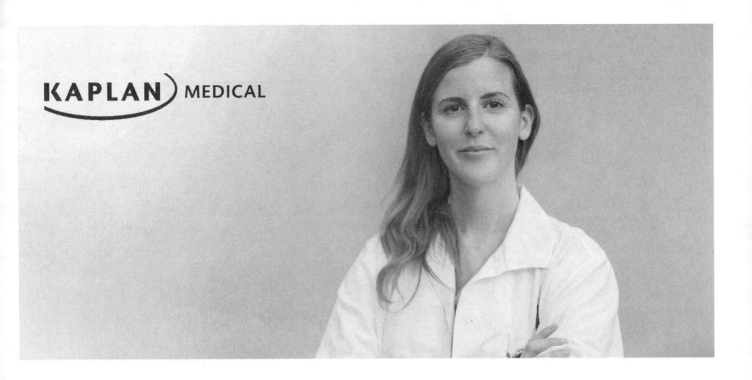

KAPLAN MEDICAL

Improve your odds of matching.

Meet our medical advisors

Our medical advisors know every exam and every part of the medical residency application process. They will be able to guide you on your course of study and better map your U.S. residency.

Discuss your:

- USMLE® study plan
- Qbank and NBME® performance
- Exam readiness
- Residency application timeline

Visit kaplanmedical.com/**medicaladvising**